A Guide to Somatic OMing*

*Things Women Have Taught Me ...
Volume I

Alutha Zatoichi Jamancar

A Guide to Somatic OMing

Copyright © 2018 Alutha Jamancar.
All rights reserved.

Printing
1

A Guide to Somatic OMing

DEDICATION ::

To Nicole Daedone ... for creating the OM Model, and for putting her brilliance, her vision, and her shadow so boldly on display.

To GL ... for pointing me towards OM.

To the Warehouse crew ... for daring to try some amazing ideas on while staying vulnerable and open in community ... for all of us to learn from.

To my research partners ... especially NVH, CC, SB, & BB ... women who patiently showed me how very little I knew.

And to women around the world ... your time is now ... your orgasm, voice, and wisdom are beholden to no one.

A Guide to Somatic OMing

A Guide to Somatic OMing

"A woman has the right to have her clitoris stroked by a trained, willing partner of her choosing ... and then get up, and go about her day ... with no strings attached, owing nothing."

— *A Clitoris Manifesto*

A Guide to Somatic OMing

TABLE OF CONTENTS ::

DEDICATION ::	3
TABLE OF CONTENTS ::	6
PREFACE ::	8
DISCLAIMERS ::	11
PART 1	13
OVERVIEW ::	14
... 1 :: What Is OM? ::	14
... 2 :: A Brief History of OM ::	16
... 3 :: The Warehouse Era ::	18
... 4 :: 'Classic' OM ::	20
... 5 :: Somatic OMing ::	21
... 6 :: Other Flavors of OM ::	22
... 7 :: The Soma ::	23
... 8 :: Gender ::	24
INTRODUCTION ::	25
:: Thumbnail History of OM ::	27
CLASSIC OM ::	29
:: Intro to Classic OM ::	29
:: About OM 'Levels' ::	30
:: Classic OM Overview ::	32
:: Introduction ::	33
:: The OM Container ::	35
:: The Nest ::	40
:: Communications ::	42
:: The Basic Practice ::	56
:: The Pussy / Anatomy ::	69
:: Orgasm ::	72
:: Community ::	76
:: OM Principles ::	97

:: OM Concepts ::	106
:: Guidance ::	122
:: Energy Patterns & Cycles ::	137
PART 2	**145**
THE MISSING 10% ::	**146**
What is a 'Clean Code' Version of OM? ::	**146**
What is 'the Missing 10%'? ::	**146**
Introducing Somatic OMing ::	**151**
An Analysis of Somatic OMing Culture ::	**153**
Soma & OM ::	154
Veritas & OM ::	156
Agency & OM ::	158
Games & OM ::	160
Shadow & OM ::	162
Mythos & OM ::	164
Mastery & OM ::	166
Tribe & OM ::	168
The 8 Cups Metaphor for the Soma	170
Orgasm & OM ::	172
Numina & OM ::	174
Identity & OM ::	176
Planet & OM ::	178
:: What's Next ::	180
:: Paths to OMing ::	181
:: Afterword ::	185
APPENDICES	**187**
:: A Clitoris Manifesto ::	188
:: The Best OM Training Going Forward ::	190
:: About the Author ::	196
:: The Design of This Book ::	199
:: The Desire & Request Distinction ::	201
:: OM Lexicon ::	203

PREFACE ::

A New Beginning ...

In the time since I set out to write this book, things – in the larger world and the world of OM (Orgasmic Meditation) – have been shifting at a breakneck pace. Since the complex social and political landscape I was writing for will likely be utterly transformed soon, I have simplified this [first] book.

I learned to OM in its golden era, the Warehouse period (2006 – 2008). I call that version of OM ... Classic OM. This work will cover some fundamentals of Classic OM. And it will cover some of the deeper practices of [Classic] OM that I fear may be lost soon to current OM practitioners.

During the Warehouse era, we came within 90% of developing a full, clean code version of OM. (By clean code version, I mean a version free of somatic viruses or malware.) I will lay out what [part of] the remaining 10% would / might look like. That 'full' version would offer people an unprecedented opportunity to develop their core communication skills and their skills in building and sourcing communities. I will [begin to] describe that 'full' version of OM here ... and have labeled it 'Somatic OMing.'

I have built a methodology called TGV (The Gaia Vedas) that I will use to explore [some of] the deeper aspects of Somatic OMing.

This work will not include everything I know about Classic OM. Nor is it intended to be an exhaustive introduction to Somatic OMing. Both will be covered in [more] depth in separate future works. This work is intended to convey what I mean by Somatic OMing and give existing OMers some ideas on how to deepen their practice and strengthen their communities.

* * *

A Guide to Somatic OMing

To OMers …

I realize that some you are just fine with your OM practice how it is. And that's awesome! This book is partially intended for those OMers I encountered over the last decade … who want detailed information about how to take their practice deeper. And for those interested in just OMing … part one of this book is focused on capturing and sharing elements of Classic OM.

* * *

Much of this book existed first as a collection of online blog entries on Facebook. Since readers tend to hop around online, there is some repetition of some content elements to aid in nonlinear browsing / reading. For consistency's sake, those repetitions have been maintained in both the ebook and paperback editions. (A Facebook Page with the weblinks from this book can be found here https://www.facebook.com/notes/somatic-oming/links-for-the-paperback-edition/1686839714758492/ or in this short link … https://tinyurl.com/yak99gml .)

* * *

The Soma & the Narratives

The body – or as I'll call it from this point on … the soma – is capable of accessing a huge variety of somatic addresses … or as they are more commonly known, 'altered states.' The practice of OM is an unusually potent and robust resource for discovering new somatic addresses and exploring existing ones.

We use narratives – stories – to order our world and make sense of our experiences. OM is essentially a collection of accumulated narratives that we use to create a particular physical and energetic shared practice.

A Guide to Somatic OMing

This book will revisit / review some of the core narratives of OM, particularly some from its peak expression in the Warehouse years ... and introduce some new narratives for the reader to consider and evaluate. The new narratives for OM that I will offer are ... new ways to 'order' your experience in and around OMing. They are just stories. You get to decide whether they have relevance and value ... as you go about weaving the larger narratives of your existence.

Good luck.

* * *

A Guide to Somatic OMing

DISCLAIMERS ::

Some Disclaimers & Advisories For This Book ...

OMing (participating in the practice of Orgasmic Meditation) is a wellness practice. If you are physically unwell or have chronic mental health issues, please consult your physician before undertaking OMing for any other challenging or stressful activity. OM partners are not trained to support people with serious physical, emotional, or mental health issues. Have a frank conversation with new partners about managing existing limitations or restrictions. Remember the principles of Informed Consent ("safeporting") and Right Range.

This is not an 'entry-level' book on OM and OMing. Readers will be presumed to have a direct, personal understanding of OM and OMing to use as a point of reference. This means they may have been explicitly trained in how to OM, or read the book, "Slow Sex," or read the chapter on Sex in "The 4-Hour Body" ... and have OMed successfully at least a handful of times.

OM is a sexual activity between consenting adults ... and is subject to the safety, security, and health 'Best Practices' of ... discretion, caution, evaluation, and vetting of partners, coaches, teachers, locations, etc.

Never OM while high. It places an unworkable burden on your OM partners ... as their physiology / body / soma attempts to track and mirror your physiology.

The OM model that has been taught has varied – slightly or largely – over the years. In general ... all variations (with a few exceptions) that have been taught by official, credentialed teachers or coaches ... may be assumed to be valid. Check with your local (or online) OM community if you think something is 'off,' out-of-date, or incorrect. Contact OneTaste to find out what the latest OM model consists of.

This book is a public discussion of the safety, security, health, and well-being

A Guide to Somatic OMing

issues of a 2-person meditative and sexual practice centered around women's sexuality. In the current political climate it is essential to continue to foster public discussions about how best to support women's sexuality and safety. This book may not reflect or describe the current OM model as privately offered by OneTaste. Please contact OneTaste for info on their current OM-related products and services (P&S) and for their latest official description of the OM model ... as offered in their P&S.

* * *

PART 1

OVERVIEW ::

... 1 :: What Is OM? ::

OM (short for 'Orgasmic Meditation') is a meditative practice that was created circa July 2004, primarily by Nicole Daedone, with support from Robert Kandell. Orgasmic Meditation or 'OM' for short ... is a two-person partnered sexual meditation with particular structures, distinctions, terminology, agreements, and set communication rituals. Over a time frame of 15 minutes ... a 'stroker' (person of any gender) ever-so-gently strokes the upper left-hand quadrant of a female 'strokee's' clitoris.

The practice of OM is designed to support women's empowerment around their agency, sexuality, orgasm, voice, and expression.

The practice of OM has been taught since about 2007 primarily by OneTaste, a company founded by Nicole and Robert, ... and to a lesser degree by graduates of Coaching Programs that OneTaste has offered over the last 8 years.

An OM is considered one complete [15-minute] cycle of this practice.

Although a few sections are out-of-date, Nicole Daedone's 2011 book, "Slow Sex," includes a good overview of the practice of OM and its associated philosophy. OneTaste has an extensive collection of videos explaining OM – many with Nicole Daedone speaking – on YouTube. OM has its own culture, mythology, history, lineage, shadow, jargon, champions, and critics. (See Wikipedia for more on Orgasmic Meditation, OneTaste, Nicole Daedone.) OM culture is separate and distinct from OneTaste culture. This book will focus on OM culture.

A Guide to Somatic OMing

OM is a sexual activity between consenting adults. It is not 'sex.' It represents a new category (at least in the West) of sexual activity, with its own limits, constraints, and agreements.

OM is not ... foreplay, an excuse to 'hit on' women, a PUA (pickup artist) technique, or connected to Tantra in any way.

* * *

... 2 :: A Brief History of OM ::

Nicole Daedone created OM in July 2004, after researching clitoris-stroking techniques for a number of years through Morehouse ("DOing") and Welcomed Consensus. She and Robert Kandell started the Urban Retreat Center in San Francisco at roughly the same time, where courses in – and related to – how to OM were first developed, field-tested, and marketed. In the summer of 2006, a residence was created nearby the Center in a converted warehouse space. This residence was designed to house 40+ OM researchers-in-residence. This experiment went from June 2006 til July 2008. Over the course of those 2 years, about a dozen of us were there for the duration. Other residents came and went ... with some part-time residents, some full-time residents, and a few 'guest' residents (via the Urban Monk Program). The first prototype for what eventually became the CP (Coaching Program) was held in the summer of 2007 and was called the Teacher Training Intensive.

There were about 5 core OM-related courses during the Warehouse Era ... most of them were either day-long or lasted a full weekend. Those courses and the volume of information they covered ... were an essential foundation of our Warehouse Era OM practice – what I am calling in this book, 'Classic' OM.

After the Warehouse Era was terminated in 2008, Nicole focused on simplifying the teaching of OM, in an effort to bring it into the mainstream. Over the following years, several OMX programs were created (a kind of mega-weekend-workshop for OMers, the OM Coaching Program (CP) was initiated, OM Houses and Affiliates were experimented with (and discarded). Several attempts to create training for 'male OMs' were tried, and shelved each time (they were found to encroach on / undermine traditional OMs). Sex Magic, 'Orgasmic Businesses,' Taboo Programs, 'OM & God' programs, and semi-arranged marriages ... came and went.

There have been to date 2 books with substantial information about how – and why – to OM: "Slow Sex," by Nicole Daedone in the spring of 2011, and "The

A Guide to Somatic OMing

4-Hour Body," by Timothy Ferriss (Dec 2010). Nicole's book covers the foundations of OM in detail, and Tim's book has an excellent chapter on OM.* (*Use gloves when OMing.)

In addition, Nicole gave a Ted Talk entitled, "Orgasm: The Cure for Hunger in the Western Woman" in 2011.

In 2017, Nicole announced that she had sold her interest in OneTaste, and in 2018 she announced that she had retired from teaching.

The new owners of OneTaste have made a number of changes and reforms to the curriculum. As of the date I write this, live OM coaching has been discontinued.

* * *

... 3 :: The Warehouse Era ::

The Warehouse Era is June 2006 til July 2008. This was the period when 40+ OM 'researchers-in-residence,' under the direct guidance of the founder of OM, Nicole Daedone, tried out her ideas, theories, and experiments ... about how best to transmit OM to the world-at-large.

The Warehouse Era of OM was an experimental community of 40+ people ... living together in a converted warehouse ... researching female orgasm, OM, connection, and intimacy. The Warehouse – as we called it – was situated in the SOMA District on Folsom Street in San Francisco. It was the brainchild of the creator of OM ... Nicole Daedone. Over those 2 years, we tested out many of her theories, ideas, and whims ... in the areas of OMing, sex, and intimacy. We learned a lot. Some of us blossomed. Others got pretty messed up. More than a few residents ended up being both.

We learned a lot. It was an abundance of data ... of lessons. To my surprise – although it was obscured by chaos, dead ends, false starts, and dramas – we got 90% of the way to a really powerful new model for human dynamics. We were *so* close. The last 10% eluded us ... and then ... with the closing of the Warehouse ... things turned to muck.

After the Warehouse experiment ended, the culture of OM – a bit rough but still relatively clean – began to be conflated and confused with the evolving commercial OM training institutions (COTI) culture.

In the years after the closing of the Warehouse, I have patiently and quietly advocated for OM, and for more transparency and responsibility by the COTIs which arose in the post-Warehouse era. When I was asked why I was so dogged, so persistent, I explained that I had appreciation for OM and that I had projects planned that depended on OM thriving ... and on the development of what I called a "clean code version of OM." For my projects, I needed a *lot* of people trained in a clean code version of OM.

A Guide to Somatic OMing

By "clean code" I mean free of the corporate malware ("FOMO", etc.) and viruses that had begun appearing around certain OM trainings and OM training promotions. The malware and viruses messed with people's heads … while OMing was simultaneously working to clear those same heads.

Over the last couple of years, COTIs have begun introducing some reforms. They also have drastically scaled back the actual methodology for transmitting (training) OM.

So … I am left with setting a new course … starting with the release of this book. It is a testament / love letter to my fellow Warehouse residents. Thank you.

* * *

... 4 :: 'Classic' OM ::

For the purposes of this work, I will be focusing on the version of OM used during the Warehouse Era, which I am calling 'Classic OM.' This represents, in my view, the richest period of OM knowledge and training thus far.

* * *

... 5 :: Somatic OMing ::

Once I lay out significant markers for Classic OM, I will introduce an extension of Classic OM, which I am calling Somatic OMing. Somatic OMing represents the lessons I have plumbed while doing Classic OM. It represents the deeper practice that I have encountered during my OMing practice.

* * *

... 6 :: Other Flavors of OM ::

Over the 14 years of OM's existence, OM has been taught in classes that have lasted as long as a weekend or as little as a few hours. People have been instructed in how to OM in classes that concluded with [optional] group OMs ... or they have learned how to OM with private instructions via a certified personal OM Coach ... or they have just had an experienced (or semi-experienced) OMer 'show them how it's done.' In more than a few cases, people have learned how to OM by cobbling together instructions from books ("Slow Sex" or "The 4-Hour Body") and / or watching a few of the videos up on YouTube (from either Nicole Daedone or OneTaste). All these people are OMers and they all OM. However, their knowledge of the basic OM Model itself and OM culture more broadly will vary ... widely. Since an up-to-date public description of the current OM Model is at present unavailable, there are a lot of (mostly minor) variations in how OM is actually practiced.

This book is an attempt to reign in the differing versions / 'flavors' of OM ... by creating a common frame of reference ("Classic OM") for OMers to have useful conversations around. The intention of this book isn't to have all OMers practicing Classic OM. It is to allow OMers to understand – using Classic OM as a jumping off point for discussions – what variation of OM they *are* practicing ... and how it relates, connects, and differs ... from other versions-in-the-wild. (And this book alone won't do the trick. I have more to write about Classic OM ... to effectively meet this need.)

* * *

... 7 :: The Soma ::

The soma is the concept that the body (or soma) is the seat or nexus of consciousness. In this model Cortex [cortex-based] Consciousness is considered a subset of the much larger Soma Consciousness. This a new distinction to OM that I will be introducing with the model of Somatic OMing.

When I use the word 'somatic,' I'm referring to "information or patterns held or present in the soma (or 'body')."

* * *

... 8 :: Gender ::

A Note About Gender ::

OM was expressly created as a practice to support empowering women around their voice, expression, orgasm, and sexuality. Although we had some women stroking women (and getting a lot out of that!), Warehouse Era (Classic OM) OM training focused in particular on the challenge of retraining women (strokees) and men (strokers) around particular archaic cultural norms, expectations, and limitations.

Since OM was created, there has been an explosion of awareness around gender … and gender narratives, agency expressions, and language. The landscape is still fluid and evolving. Since anyone of any gender expression may act as a stroker in an OM, I will adopt the gender-neutral language of 'they' instead of the original 'he' for the stroker position. After much reflection, I will maintain the use of 'woman' / 'she' as the person being stroked ("strokee"). A major cultural shift is occurring as I write this, and women are reclaiming part of their power and expression. It is premature, as a result, to move on and reduce OM to a "woman-free space"(via exclusive use of gender-neutral language) … in the face of such courage and struggles.

So I will be using 'she' for strokee … and 'they' for stroker. I will include sections addressing the unique perspective, challenges, and [potential] gifts of … women stroking women … and men stroking women. Those sections will use relevant gender language.

A later volume of this project may dive more deeply into parsing OM into updated gendering language and distinctions. For now, women will continue to hold center stage.

* * *

INTRODUCTION ::

OM stands for 'Orgasmic Meditation.' The model for OM was established by Nicole Daedone, with assistance from Rob Kandell, in July 2004. In the 14 years since its inception, the central model of OM has varied slightly, as the lead proponents tweaked and tinkered with it. More importantly, how it was transmitted (aka, OM training), has varied widely over even a few years' time. The richest OM training offered thus far (as of the date of this book) was – in my opinion – the period from June 2006 to July 2008, nicknamed the Warehouse Era.

For the purposes of this work, I will be focusing on the version of OM used during the Warehouse Era, which I am calling 'Classic OM.'

Once I lay out significant markers for Classic OM, I will introduce an extension of Classic OM, which I am calling Somatic OMing. Somatic OMing represents the lessons I have plumbed while doing Classic OM. It represents the deeper practice that I encountered during my OMing practice.

I am writing this book and covering these topics because a lot of deep, accumulated wisdom that was built up during the Warehouse years is, I fear, in danger of being lost. So, while the condensed survey of Classic OM I am including in this book is not complete, I hope it will serve as a start to capturing a very rich body of experience, one that I have had the privilege of participating in. Additionally, for years I have been navigating OM discussions and conversations with a deep reservoir of intuited learnings – based on my OM experience and the experiences others have shared with me – and I am surfacing and languaging those accumulated learnings and making them available as an integrated body of knowledge called 'Somatic OMing.' As with Classic OM, the description of Somatic OMing in this book will be a beginning one. It will take me longer and more volumes to adequately cover either Classic OM or Somatic OMing. But in the meantime, this work can serve as a resource for OMers wishing to take their practice deeper.

My descriptions of Classic OM and Somatic OMing aren't gospel, just one person's descriptions. That being said, I had the privilege of living full time in the Warehouse community for two very full years (July 2006 – July 2008). In that short time I did over 2000 OMs. I assisted in some of the core classes we produced to support OMers in their practice. I received a lot of excellent coaching and feedback from a lot of veteran women OMers around how to deepen my [OM] practice. Which I took to heart. And I attended a lot of group OMs – particularly our community's morning group OMs.

That is a lot of information I was exposed to. My OMing began in a community of 40+ other OMers, and that *greatly* accelerated and deepened my development as a stroker.

And this book is – in part – a way of saying thank you to my Warehouse gang … by sharing with you what I discovered (and what was shared with me by other OMers) along the way.

This book is not perfect, but it is a start. Experienced OMers need to write more books about OM … and share with others in the OM community – through stories, discoveries, and art – what we have encountered along the way. We need to discover and pool our Best Practices – and out any Worst Practices we encounter.

More than ever … the world could benefit from having clean, public access to OM.

* * *

A Guide to Somatic OMing

:: Thumbnail History of OM ::

Nicole Daedone studied clit stroking (it was called 'DOing') at Morehouse and Welcomed Consensus prior to creating the OM Model in 2004. Victor Baranco was one of her mentors. She oversaw 3 'houses' in Brisbane, whose dozen or so residents explored and researched partnered orgasm practices.

In the early 2000s, Nicole led the creation of an 'Urban Retreat Center' in downtown San Francisco, where [some of] the first OM courses took place. In spring of 2006, that enterprise was expanded to include a 40+ person residence dedicated to researching sex, orgasm, and OM – with a specific focus on exploring and supporting women's orgasm, leadership, and expression. That residence was an old warehouse that volunteers (many of them future residents) helped convert into a spartan, open-space, co-ed living quarters, which we called, simply, the Warehouse. The peak of the Warehouse Years was probably the 3-month Teacher Training Program (TTP), which Nicole offered to select students in the summer of 2007. Up until then, Nicole was the sole teacher for all of the major courses we offered – including the Intro to OM Courses. Smaller evening programs were managed by her student teachers – all of whom were women. TTP was intended to train other women (and men) to be able to teach the major [OM-related] courses … independent of Nicole.

After Nicole (via her business partner, Robert Kandell) declared the Warehouse Experiment over in July 2008, there was a transition period of about 18 months. Nicole kept a small core of students with her for the next phase. The rest of the residents were thanked and moved on. At the end of that period (roughly), a nearby small hotel had been procured and reconditioned to serve as a new "OM-friendly" residence. The new building was simply called by its street address, "1080." The large open communal spaces of the Warehouse were replaced by small rooms (with actual doors that closed!) occupied by either one or two persons. OM courses and some non-OM courses were produced by OneTaste (OT), and students and teachers often lived in 1080. After a few successful years, 1080 was shut down.

Also after the end of the Warehouse Experiment, the first in a series of months-long [OM] Coaching Programs (CPs) were offered. CPs originally offered training in OM and OM culture, and some basic certification. The course content of the actual CPs and the certification specifics varied widely over the years. Currently the 16th CP is wrapping up. Each CP graduated a number of its students, some of whom elected to pursue certification, others content to simply have had the training. When someone indicates that they are an 'OM Coach,' most of the time they are indicating they took part in (and completed) one or more CPs.

Of note are the 2 OMX events (2013 & 2014). These events brought together hundreds of OMers to a weekend of OM-related (and non OM-related) programs ... and a number of large group OMs. The OMX events represent a peak of OM-in-the-world, in the post-Warehouse Era. The 2015 OMX was cancelled.

Over the last decade, OT experimented with different variations of local 'centers' in major cities. For a while there were franchise cities, affiliate cities, and outpost cities. Currently there are a handful of major cities that offer regular OM training, although that may be in flux at this moment.

In 2017, Nicole Daedone retired from leading OM and OneTaste, and sold OneTaste to new owners. The new owners have made a number of changes, including some needed reforms. They also ended live OM coaching.

* * *

CLASSIC OM ::

:: Intro to Classic OM ::

This work is designed for people who have been trained in how to OM and who have OMed at least a few times. It is intended as a resource for them to take their practices deeper.

For the purposes of this work, I will be focusing on the version of OM used during the Warehouse Era (2006 – 2008), which I am calling 'Classic OM.' When I learned to OM in April 2006, the training that was offered specifically to support and deepen one's OM practice consisted of a handful of courses … most of which were a full day or a weekend of training each. After the Warehouse experiment's end was announced in July 2008, the trainings related directly to OM were scaled back significantly. Principles, distinctions, and exercises were dropped or shelved. Warehouse Era OMing was the peak iteration (in my opinion) of the OM Model. Subsequent offerings lacked many of the components that I found essential in my OM practice. For this reason, I identify the Warehouse-era OM Model as the Classic OM Model.

***

[Classic] OM is fundamentally about truthtelling, an energy-based practice, and a community-based practice.

***

:: About OM 'Levels' ::

The Basic OM ::

The Basic OM is a 2-person meditative practice where a woman has her clitoris stroked with *very, very* light strokes by a second person (of any gender) wearing gloves ... for a fixed 15-minute time period.

Making a clean request for an OM — and handling the responses (the 'yes'es' and 'no's') gracefully – is considered part of an OM.

Note that the distinction between 'basic' and 'advanced' OM weren't formalized in any consistent way during (or after) the Warehouse era. Instead, part of the process of identifying and describing Classic OM entails languaging and codifying *how we as a community handled different kinds of OM questions and experiences.* There was – generally – a subtle but noticeable shift in how we addressed advanced OM topics ... even though we often resisted calling them advanced. The Warehouse community / researchers followed the founder's preference for avoid languaging – or establishing – OM grades or levels. They existed. We just avoided formalizing them. I am attempting to put them into language now ... so that the distinctions and lessons we so carefully acquired aren't lost.

Advanced Practice ::

After completing between 300 and 1000 OMs ... and developing a solid practice (both strokees & strokers: good communication habits, good container holding, an increase in range of and ability to hold sensation), some OMers choose to pursue certain advanced OM practices. These include: Group OMs, a series of optional OM exercises, introital strokes, and women-stroking-women. Note: advanced practice requests should be initiated *only* by the woman (strokee) for *at least* the first 25 OMs done together.

A Guide to Somatic OMing

Research OMs ::

An even more advanced topic are 'Research OMs.' Generally, in a research OM, *experienced OMers* will decide together ahead of an OM – or string of OMs – to take one aspect of OM and explore it with their attention / awareness. They might research upstrokes by doing 10 upstrokes for every downstroke, calling out when they feel themselves disconnecting (only one partner should do this per OM), intentionally focus on 'going over' (climaxing), or other topics.

When the OM is all done – frames and all – the 2 partners get together and compare notes. This is a structured way for two experienced OMers, both with a solid OM practice, to carefully expand their range and knowledge.

* * *

The next section is a brief overview of Classic OM elements. The elements are described by using discrete entries. Feel free to share them with other OM practitioners. The overview is neither complete, nor exhaustive. Its purpose is to serve as common frame of reference for the reader going forward. As I introduce core concepts of Somatic OMing, I may point back to some of the sections on Classic OM to illustrate various points.

* * *

:: Classic OM Overview ::

:: Introduction ::

:: The OM Container ::

:: The Nest ::

:: Communications ::

:: The Basic Practice ::

:: The Pussy / Anatomy ::

:: Orgasm ::

:: Community ::

:: OM Principles ::

:: OM Concepts ::

:: Guidance ::

:: Strokes ::

:: Energy Patterns & Cycles ::

A Guide to Somatic OMing

:: Introduction ::

ORGASMIC MEDITATION (OM)

This meditative practice was created circa July 2004, primarily by Nicole Daedone, with support from Robert Kandell. Orgasmic Meditation or 'OM' for short ... is a two-person partnered sexual meditation with particular structures, distinctions, terminology, agreements, and set rituals. Over a time frame of 15 minutes ... a 'stroker' (person of any gender) ever-so-gently strokes the upper left-hand quadrant of a female 'strokee's' clitoris.

The practice of OM has been taught since 2007 primarily by OneTaste, a company founded by Nicole and Robert, ... and to a lesser degree by graduates of Coaching Programs that OneTaste has offered over the last 8 years.

Although sections are out-of-date, Nicole Daedone's 2011 book, "Slow Sex," includes a good overview of the practice of OM and its associated philosophy. OneTaste has an extensive collection of videos explaining OM – many with Nicole Daedone speaking – on YouTube. Another good introduction to OM can be found in Tim Ferris' book, "The 4-Hour Body," in the chapter on ___.

OM has its own culture, mythology, history, lineage, shadow, jargon, champions, and critics.

(See Wikipedia for more on Orgasmic Meditation, OneTaste, Nicole Daedone.)

This book will cover elements of OM taught during the peak of OM research, the Warehouse Era (June 2006 – July 2008). The 'Warehouse' was a nickname for an experimental community of amateur researchers researching sex, intimacy, and OM. That version of OM will be called 'Classic OM' in this book, to distinguish it from later versions offered with differing training models over the last decade. For information on the latest iteration of OM and OM Training, please contact OneTaste.*

(*This is not a recommendation or endorsement.)

OMs can be private (just 2 people ... or 2 people and a coach), or there can be [scheduled] group OMs ... typically referred to as OM Circles.

OM Etiquette: there is surprisingly a lot to learn about OM culture, etiquette, and communication rituals. Indeed, one of the strongest contributions of OM ... is the retraining of long-seated miscues, prejudices, and restrictive superstitions of western culture. OM isn't just "pussy-stroking" – there are dozens (and probably have been hundreds over the millennia) of pussy-stroking models / systems. What makes OM so potent and useful in this 21st century ... is the encompassing social model (culture) is a fully formed alternative – and vast improvement – to the sinking quagmire of today's meta-culture (aka, "the west").

OM etiquette includes distinguishing cleanly between desire and request, sharing clean frames, 'holding space' for someone or some group ... and much, much more. [link to full essay later.]

So OM etiquette isn't just a 'nicety,' afterthought, or an embellishment – it is the branches of the tree itself.

You stroke her pussy ... show some respect.

* * *

:: The OM Container ::

Container

The OM Container serves as a bedrock for the entire practice. It was largely defined by 2006, and has changed in minor ways over the years as a result of attempts to make refinements.

The OM Container is basically a set of agreements about what—exactly—happens in an OM and how it should happen. It creates – reliably – a formal, yet limbic way for two practitioners to safely connect. And its consistency permits OM practitioners around the world to connect with strangers who they may have barely met and have an OM together.

The concept of container—and more importantly, the limbic lessons seasoned practitioners acquire over the course of their practice—translates in *really* useful ways to "real" life. The trickiest part is often just recognizing the [social] containers we encounter in our day-to-day lives.

A copy of the most current version of the OM Container document has been available in PDF form in recent years. (Note: slightly different versions of the OM Container "Official" PDF are floating around. Always checkin with new partners and review the expected steps to OM.) The most recent version as of the date of this writing is version 1.2.2 and is from 2017. (You can find the link for the OM Container doc in the OneTaste.us website footer.)

OM Jargon

The following are some instances of relevant OM jargon or slang. The entries are intended to be freestanding, so feel free to jump around … or read them in order.

Keep a Strong [OM] Container: OM is a practice designed to source and empower women around their sexuality and expression. OM has a 'container' ... consisting of an explicit set of agreements and practices ... that allow a woman to open her sex, be stroked for 15 minutes, and then get up and go about her day – without any hassles. "Keeping a strong container" means simply knowing and honoring those agreements and sticking to the structure and form of the OM as designed. It doesn't mean hitting on the woman, making out with her, or "poaching" in the container. It definitely doesn't mean manipulating a partner ... in order to weaken or collapse those agreements (and thus weakening or collapsing the container). (See entries above for "Container" and "Collapsing the Container.")

Honoring the [OM] Container ... is a way of honoring the woman.

Maintain a Clean Container: the "container" here is the 'social container' of OM – the set of agreements, distinctions, and practices / rituals that make up a proper OM. (See the terms above ... "Collapsing the Container" and "Container" and "Leaky Container.")

'Maintain a Clean Container' ... means to have and maintain a skilled awareness of those agreements, distinctions, and practices / rituals ... and to follow them conscientiously. If an OM container step is skipped or a container agreement is broken ... that is called "breaking the container."

(The 2017 OT Container document (PDF) is a key reference source for OMers.)

Tight Container: this means keeping the agreements of the OM container – and avoiding doing any "wriggling" or 'sneaking' around the edges. (See the terms "container" and "strong container.")

No [Container] Poaching: this refers almost exclusively to male strokers who have the bad habit of "pulling for" more intimacy by using subtle container breaks and energy leaks ... to persuade their female strokees ... to "give him a little sugar." It typically occurs in or around the OM nest ... but it builds on the underlying OMing relationship … so it can also occur elsewhere, implicitly leveraging the OM relationship.

This is straight up sleazy manipulation … with one goal: to get more 'gestures of affection / intimacy / sex' … than a woman actually wants to give. It is at its best … an integrity failure … and at its worst … an instance of predatory behavior.

If your stroker takes adjustments well / gracefully … and if they demonstrate that they are trainable … some small errors may be tolerated. However, if a 'new' stroker keeps making the same – or similar – container breaks, assume they don't really 'want' to change. Toss them back into the pool … and pass on your experience (privately) to other women.

Steer clear of OM Container Poachers.

Breaking the Container: the "container" is the set of agreements and practices that constitute the "game" (or 'practice') of OM. "Breaking" the container means breaking the foundational set of agreements … that allow an OM to take place. A container "break" can be willful or accidental. In the beginning of a stroker's OM practice … they may make a lot of unintentional mistakes to start with.

And … some strokers (most often men) will break a container intentionally … and lie about it or gaslight their partners if they are called on it. (And there are some veteran strokers who pull this … so head's up.) They should be dumped until they are retrained and vetted – or banned within a community, if they are unwilling to play nicely.

Unfortunately, the institutions responsible for OM training have been historically messy in teaching the OM Container. As a result, it is possible for 8 people (new to one another) to come to a group OM … and for them to have 8 slightly *different* maps for what constitutes "the official OM container." It is … therefore … imperative that **when 2 people OM together for the first time, they do a thorough review of what each "thinks" a 'normal' OM consists of.**

A Guide to Somatic OMing

Getting on the same page is key. When in doubt, defer to the person with the pussy [that will be stroked]. Checkin with veteran OMers (especially women) in online or real-world OM communities for guidance, suggestions, and "best practices."

Container Break: an instance in which one of the core agreements underlying the OM container is broken (whether intentionally or not intentionally). Navigating container breaks – and setting firm boundaries – is part of the practice (but shouldn't become the centerpiece).

Choose partners wisely. Get good OM training.

Collapsing the Container: this usually refers to one or both partners ... "switching" post-OM (or for established couples ... mid-OM) into sexual contact. Across the board – including with married couples – this a bad idea. And usually ... the woman (even if she initiates it) pays for it. It takes a long time for the deeper parts of a woman's body ... to trust *her,* ... let alone a male partner. A part of creating the space for OM ... is making sure that the usual "deals" and energetic "sales" that accompany almost all contemporary sexual pairings are off the table. That means ... if a woman OMs with her stroker ... afterwards she *owes* them NOTHING.

By collapsing the container ... that "horsetrading" makes its way into the OM space ... and suddenly ... next time, he's just ... "oh, honey ... let's just makeout. It was so much fun last time ...." And quality time [OM] with a woman's pussy is suddenly gone for her.

Generally, even for married couples,, there should be a firm and clean end to the OM ... and at *least* a 15 minute "cooling down" period ... so that you are not "leaching" off the turn-on from the OM. And – if you are that desperate to use OM as a jumpstart for your sex – you have other issues. Get *real* sex coaching / support. (See AASECT for **actual** certified sex coaches, therapists, and teachers. https://www.aasect.org/)

A Guide to Somatic OMing

Leaky Container: this implies one or both OM partners is 'soft' or collapses easily around core OM [container] agreements. (See the entry for "Container" above.) A container can only be 'leaky' if one or both parties are 'soft' on actually maintaining it.

* * *

:: The Nest ::

NEST

The nest is central to the OM. Physically, it is a combination of padding (blankets and / or yoga pads), cushions / pillows ... together with a quiet, comfortable, well-lit physical space ... that is confidently private for the set-up, duration, and wrap-up of the OM. No surprises, no unexpected guests.

Energetically, it is a safe space ... which the stroker looks after (safeguards) ... so that the woman who is being stroked ... can relax her vigilance center ... and sink deeply into her orgasm. The stroker has the strokee's back. If anything surprising occurs in the vicinity ... the stroker names it ... in a way to reassure the strokee. Only in unusual circumstances should the strokee find it necessary to "get up and handle something" (like something urgent with a child). (In over 2500 OMs, my strokee has never had to interrupt her OM.) Creating and maintaining this space ... for the duration of an OM ... is excellent practice in setting clean boundaries ... and communicating clearly (safeporting) your household members.

(More can be found on the nest here.)

OM JARGON

The following are some instances of relevant OM jargon or slang.

Nest Etiquette: there are some basic guidelines to being in or around an OM nest ... during OMs. These guidelines are a way of being courteous and respectful ... in [socially] unusual circumstances. Some nest etiquette may be considered global / universal ... while others may be used only locally. If you travel and OM someplace new with local OMers ... be sure to ask what their local customs do / do not include.

A Guide to Somatic OMing

Entering the Nest: Generally, the woman enters the nest first ... gets herself situated, makes requests and adjustments to her pillows. Her stroker then sits down and adjusts their pillows / cushions / support. If at all possible ... don't step over the woman. (Her body will likely tense involuntarily – which is the opposite of your goal.) The stroker makes any needed adjustments to the OM towel position – after safeporting the woman. Once they are settled ... the stroker reaches over to arrange the lube, timer, and gloves. The stroker may do a final pre-OM checkin with the woman ... often just making brief eye contact and asking, "You good?" Upon confirmation from her ... the stroker proceeds with the prepping for the start of the OM (putting gloves on, etc.).

Exiting the Nest: The OM 'nest' is where the OM takes place. After the OM is concluded ... if the nest will be left intact ... then the woman and her stroker 'exit' the nest. This language – and the distinction itself – are in support of maintaining a 'clean' OM container. The intent is not to have other activities "spill" into the OM space (the nest). The nest is for OMs only. When you are finished with the OM (and you intend to leave the nest out for future scheduled OMs), you consciously and deliberately 'exit' the OM nest / space.

Tidying Up the Nest: after an OM is completed, the OM nest may need to be tidied up and put away. (In some situations, they may need to be left out.) Leave things well in order for the next OM and the next stroker. (In general, the stroker tidies up ... unless the strokee insists on helping – or doing it herself. She may still be lingering in the afterglow of the OM. Respect that.)

Pay attention to the used OM towel ... and handle it prudently. (Don't get lube on other things.)

* * *

A Guide to Somatic OMing

:: Communications ::

Communicating is a vital part of OMing. As in many cultures, core communications have become ritualized. This means they have a structure and form that helps orient members of the culture. In this case ... OM practitioners. Here are some examples of OM-specific communications.

OM Jargon

The following are some instances of relevant OM jargon or slang.

Request an OM

There is a certain protocol to request an OM. It is designed to support women ... not having to explain or justify themselves.

If you want to OM with someone, you say, "would you like to OM?" ... or "do you want to OM?" Either person can make the request. A simple, clear, 'Yes' or 'No,' is all that is required. Women often are pressured or harassed ... to turn a 'No' into a 'Yes' in the outside world ... often by asking – if they say 'No' – "but why?!" In OM ... their 'No' is sufficient. Period. They don't owe *anyone* an explanation. (This practice is extended to other requests within OM culture, with the intention being to create a space where women's choices – and voices – are fully honored.)

It is important to note ... that if you ask a woman to OM ... and she has clearly heard you ... and doesn't reply ... that should be taken as a 'No' – and honored as such. Social pressure comes in many forms, and many women have experienced abuse and sexual assault. Your request ... does not compel a verbal answer from her. Treat her with respect ... and move on.

Phrases that are considered bad form, include ...

A Guide to Somatic OMing

- ✦ *"Can I OM you?"*
- ✦ *"Will you OM me?"*

… both of these upend the description of OM being a "partnered" practice. OM is a joint venture … requiring both people's unique contributions. It isn't "done" to anyone.

Again … this is part of creating a culture that re-trains people to honor consent and agency.

Booking (Scheduling) an OM: the process of asking to OM at some specific future time (and space), getting a 'yes,' and scheduling it.

Book a #1: in OM circles (group OMs) there are typically 2 rounds of scheduled OMs. The first one … is called "a #1" for short. 'Booking a #1' … is the process of asking for a #1 from someone (for a specific OM circle at a specific time, date, and location), getting a 'yes,' and scheduling it.

Book a #2: in OM circles (group OMs) there are typically 2 rounds of scheduled OMs. The second one … is called "a #2" for short. 'Booking a #2' … is the process of asking for a #2 from someone (for a specific OM circle at a specific time, date, and location), getting a 'yes,' and scheduling it.

Double-Booking [an OM]: this usually occurs in a group OM / OM circle context. Double-booking an OM means that you booked the same OM with two different people. You booked Tuesday's #1 OM with Maggie … then forgot about her … and booked it with Alice. Tuesday's OM circle arrives … and whoops! Somebody has to be bumped. Double-booking – while not the end of the world – is a sign of sloppiness (and disrespect). Avoid it. Have a reliable system to keep track of your OMs … and use it. (If you book an OM more than day out, do a courtesy follow-up via text or some other *discrete* channel … the day of or before your OM … confirming that you are good for the OM on _____ at ____ pm. That will gently remind them.

Strokers ... if your strokee slips up ... be graceful. You will earn points. Don't sulk, pout, or lash out ... you will lose points. Remember ... your record with one woman is your record with all women. Be impeccable, prompt, prepared, quiet, positive. Show up on time. Leave on time ... don't overstay your welcome. Many people book an OM ... and need to get on with their day.

Strokees ... the more respectful you are of your strokers' time ... the faster your stable of strokers will grow.

Safeport: Letting your partner know what you're going to do ... before you do it. Safeporting implies asking for permission, or at least giving them an opportunity to opt out. Think of it as refined form of 'heads up.'

At the start of an OM, a stroker will say ... "I'm going to touch your pussy now ...." This is the most prominent example of safeporting in an OM.

Color Codes for internal level of comfort: these are handy for shorthanding where you are at ... but only if you have confirmed (ahead of time) that your partner knows about them ... AND you have made sure you are on the same page. (Some OM trainings included them, others omitted them.)

>*Green*: Easy comfort zone, cruising.

>*Yellow*: Edge of your comfort zone / right range; challenging but doable.

>*Red*: Beyond breaking point, overwhelmed; STOP and take care of yourself.

REQUEST

In OM either person may make a request (subject to the constraints of OM Container). It is the custom in OM culture that the response be yes or no ... with no further explanation needed. The best example of this is the request to OM. Either person can ask the other, "Would you like to OM?" A simple, clear, 'Yes' or 'No,' is all that is required.* Women often are pressured or harassed ...

A Guide to Somatic OMing

to turn a 'No' into a 'Yes' in the outside world. In OM ... their 'No' is sufficient. Period. They don't owe *anyone* an explanation. This practice is extended to other requests within OM culture, with the intention being to create a space where women's choices – and voices – are fully honored.

(*It is important to note ... that if you ask a woman to OM ... and she has clearly heard you ... and doesn't reply ... that should be taken as a 'No' – and honored as such. Social pressure comes in many forms, and many women have experienced abuse and sexual assault. Your request ... does not compel a verbal answer from her. Treat her with respect ... and move on.)

(IMPORTANT: See also the FB Note on "Distinction Between Desire & Request.")

Clean Requests: a request where the person is not under pressure to give one particular response ... and where 'yes' or 'no' are both going to be accepted and honored – fully – as responses. A request that is specific and understood clearly by both parties – in the same way.

An 'unclean' request is when the requester ... is 'pulling' — subtly or not so subtly – for one response over the other.

Clean Agreements: an agreement that is reached ... where both parties are fully informed on the specific details of the agreement – and when the agreement *is* specific and concrete ... where there is no coercion / bullying / manipulative transactions ... and where 'yes' or 'no' were both going to be accepted – fully – as responses ... is a clean agreement.

Saying 'yes' to a vague agreement ... is not a clean agreement. Making an agreement while withholding intimacy is being threatened ... is not a clean agreement. Getting a 'yes' and then surreptitiously 'changing' the agreement details ... is not a clean agreement. Whining to get a 'yes' ... is not a clean agreement.

- ✦ **[a] Clean 'No':** a 'no' which is not bullied or coerced or tricked out of the person answering.

- ✦ **[a] Clean 'Yes':** a 'yes' which is not bullied or coerced or tricked out of the person answering.

Request Adjustment Strokes: the phrase 'request adjustment strokes' ... means a person is *explicitly* asking for ... suggestion or observations on how they may modify or improve 'how they are showing up.' In an OM, the woman is encouraged to request adjustments of her stroker ... if she wants them to change something (pressure, speed, location ... of the stroke). She is encouraged to make the request in a neutral voice ... so the stroker can concentrate on the actual request – and not be sidelined by any reaction they might have to the delivery of the request.

As with many elements of OM, this concept is used – among OMers – outside the nest / OM, as well. It reinforces the concepts of consent and agency. If a woman wants your advice / feedback – she'll ask for it.

Receive Adjustments: to 'receive adjustments' in an OM ... is to be given change instructions ... from the strokee, or from a person ***who has been requested*** to live coach the OM, or – far more rarely – by an *experienced* stroker. (The 'adjustments' offered by a stroker should be rare and not "pushed" on the strokee – it is her ride, her body 'leads' the OM ... never the stroker.)

Like many OM terms, this one is used in day-to-day living. It was used when people made requests or suggestions ... or more generally, presented subtle feedback ... that needed to be gently highlighted.

Clean Adjustments: [In an OM] a change may be requested by a woman (often in speed, position, or pressure of a stroke) ... or a stroker may be in an awkward sitting position in the nest and may request a change; [Outside of an OM] a request for a specific change in communication, presence, or communication style. (The concept of 'adjustments' is one of the OM principles ... that transfers nicely to the 'real' world as well.)

A Guide to Somatic OMing

A clean adjustment is specific and delivered without hooks or barbs. If you roll your eyes while you give an adjustment, that's not a clean adjustment. If you make your adjustment request with a begging voice, that's not a clean adjustment. If you piggyback a second communication onto the adjustment request ... their body will have *two* communications to respond to ... and things can go off the rails relatively easily.

Adjustable: open to trying out suggestions or following through on requests (often called in OM ... 'adjustments').

Adjustment: an adjustment is a value-neutral request for a different action. It is not an agreement that anything is wrong or bad. It allows for a strong relationship to 'what's so' to be maintained and cultural agreements to be explored and shared.

[In an OM] a change may be requested by a woman (often in speed, position, or pressure of a stroke) ... or a stroker may be in an awkward sitting position in the nest and may request a change. [outside of an OM] a request for a specific change in communication, presence, or communication style. (The concept of 'adjustments' is one of the OM principles ... that transfers nicely to the 'real' world as well.)

[a] Check-In [with your partner]: during an OM a person may ask their partner a question. "Shall I decrease the pressure?" Often the exact question is just an excuse to 'check-in' more broadly ... aka, somatically. As a stroker ... I will feel the energy in her reply ... and "feel" into her ... to get a sense of where she is. I avoid doing this [asking questions] a lot ... as it can be disruptive. Again ... there is a verbal 'check-in' ... on which a deeper 'somatic check-in' is piggybacked. My body wants to check in on where her body is at. (While knowing that her cortex mind may be at a *very* different place.) So, during a checkin, I will pay attention to her verbal response ... and also pay attention to her somatic presentation / communication: voice tone, present / disconnected, alert / bored, etc.

A Guide to Somatic OMing

Many times the somatic portion of her response will tell me volumes ... while her verbal response might be a simple, "fine...."

Again, checkins should not be overused. And it will take some people a while to get the hang of them. OMing will aid that process.

Receiving a Communication: our Warehouse OM training had a great distinction: to "receive" a communication. It basically meant ... that you "let the communication in." You didn't necessarily agree with the communication or align with it ... but you didn't block or deflect it either. You 'received' it. You got it.

In response ... you might reply, "I got it," or "I get that" ... or more generally ... "thank you."

This has value in and around OM ... because as women become more connected to their pussy / body ... a *lot* of anger / grief / sadness / rage can surface. Women both culturally and personally have had to push a lot of stuff down. When it comes back up ... it sometimes gets directed momentarily at whatever's / whoever's nearest. Being able to receive a charge-y communication without blocking it / deflecting it / taking it personally ... can come in handy for a stroker. And can be liberating for the woman on the other end.

Sensory-Specific Reports: this means avoiding judgmental language (beautiful, awful, disgusting, rapturous, etc.) as well as avoiding the use of metaphor ("it was like a butterfly") ... and sticking to concrete sensory details (color, texture, pitch, etc.) only ... when you report an experience (for example, shared about an afternoon OM you had just done). (See also the entry for Frames.)

FRAME

Frames are exchanged at the end of an OM. Frames are sensory-specific words to describe an OMer's experience at one moment in the OM ... such as temperature, texture, pressure, and vibrations. A frame contains no sexual content or use of 'naughty language.' Use of metaphor is kept to a minimum.

A Guide to Somatic OMing

The objective isn't to highlight or showcase one's poetry skills ... it is to "directly" transmit a report about the actual sensations on experienced at a moment of the OM.

The intent is twofold: first, to create a bridge between one's physical experience and one's own language, (Westerners – especially men – are chronically disconnected from their own bodies, and often lack the language to use if they actually feel something.); and second, to create a *neutral* bridge language between partners, so they can compare their experiences in safety.)Avoid words that imply status.)

Some common occurrences among newbies ... include copying frames you overhear from another couple. Don't. Own your experience. Wherever you are at is fine. The body moves at its own pace. Stop pushing it. Many [western] men report 'feeling nothing' in their bodies ... at the start of their OM practice. For my first six months of OMing, my frame 60% of the time was ... "there was a moment when I felt a slight buzzing in my stroking finger." Eventually ... my body woke up and I had a huge range of sensations to share. Because of OMing regularly and learning to share frames.

For many men especially ... feeling anything other than anger or an erection ... is unheard of. It takes time to open up that creaky box ... of actual sensations ... given how often they [may] have been blocked. Culturally, men's feelings are often labelled "Dangerous!" ... and avoided entirely. The exchange – and discipline – of frames ... is part of the process of slowly reconnecting to our bodies ... and giving voice – and validation – to our somatic / limbic experience.

OM can assist men in safely and slowly reawakening a deep connection to their own bodies – in a space of approval.

'Clean' frames means that there no 'embellishments added to the basic sensory report. Often, new OMers – especially men – will want to "impress" their partner ... with flowery, over-the-top 'frames.' Or with overtly (or covertly) sexual frames. Both can occur as thinly concealed 'pickup lines.' Guys ... you

A Guide to Somatic OMing

are not OMing to 'hump' her. You are creating a safe space for her sexuality to be explored – by her. Don't crowd her or mash [on] her or hit on her. Keep your frames sensory-specific and content-neutral. You can journal later if you need to verbalize more. Privately.

As with other OM distinctions, the concept of frames transfers well to the 'real world.' Teaching kids the concept of sharing [clean] frames … means you are giving them a tool to connect with their bodies … and language what they are *actually* feeling.

Lastly, you can always argue with (or judge) emotion-laden language ("they didn't say they loved me enough…") … while a clean report of the actual sensations you felt (aka, 'frames'), leaves really no traction for bickering or arguing. Frames can help us stay connected … in really high sensation states (ecstasy or anger).

Exchanging Frames: At the conclusion of an OM … before the nest is put away … the woman and her stroker exchange frames. Frames are sensory-specific "snapshots" of what each person experienced in their bodies … at a moment of the OM of their choosing. (See the entry on "Frames.")

Clean Frames: 'Frames' are composed of sensory-specific words to describe an OMer's experience at one moment in the OM … such as temperature, texture, pressure, and vibrations. A frame contains no sexual content or use of 'naughty language.' Avoid language conveying emotions – they can trigger social comparisons and judgements.

The intent is twofold: first, to create a bridge between one's physical experience and one's own language, (Westerners – especially men – are chronically disconnected from their bodies, and often lack the language to use *if* they actually feel something.); and second, to create *neutral* bridge language between partners, so they can compare their experiences.

'Clean' frames means that there no 'embellishments added to the basic sensory report. Avoid using metaphors … you are sharing *your* sensations, not painting a canvas. Often, new OMers – especially men – will want to "impress" their partner ... with flowery, over-the-top 'frames.' Or overtly (or covertly) sexual frames. Both can occur as thinly concealed 'pickup lines.' Guys ... you are not OMing to 'hump' her. You are creating a safe space for her sexuality to be explored – by her. Don't crowd her or hit on her. Keep your frames sensory-specific and content-neutral. You can journal later if you need to verbalize more. Privately.

Framing to Impress: Often, new OMers – especially men – will want to "impress" their partner ... with flowery, over-the-top 'frames.' Or with overtly (or covertly) sexual frames. Both can occur as thinly concealed 'pickup lines.' Guys ... you are not OMing to 'hump' her. You are creating a safe space for her sexuality to be explored – by her. Don't crowd her or hit on her. Keep your frames sensory-specific and content-neutral. You can journal later if you need to verbalize more.

"Sexual" Frames: some new OMers "dress up" their frames ... to impress their partners or to "hook" them with flattery ... or because they think that is 'how to give frames.' They may add sexual language or evocative poetic expressions.

In OM, frames are *only* composed of sensory-specific words to describe an OMer's experience at one moment in the OM ... such as temperature, texture, pressure, and vibrations. A frame contains no sexual content or use of 'naughty language.' (See earlier entries for "Frames" and "Clean Frames.")

Flower-y Frames: some new OMers "dress up" their frames ... to impress their partners ... or because they think that is 'how to give frames.' They may add sexual language or evocative poetic expressions.

Frames are composed of sensory-specific words to describe an OMer's experience at one moment in the OM ... such as temperature, texture, pressure, and vibrations. A frame contains no sexual content or use of 'naughty language.'

COACH [AN OM]

To 'coach' an OM ... means a more experienced OMer ... *__has been requested to observe an OM and chime in during the OM and offer their guidance (on one specific piece or more generally) – and has agreed to do such.__*

While there are official certified and / or trained OM coaches around, their quality and training / standards vary widely. There are people who are "official" coaches ... who have no business doing OM coaching. Your best bet is to ask around for an experienced OMer with a stellar reputation who is willing to give advice ... based on their *actual* OM experience. After that, peruse your local "official" OM coaches warily. Ask around privately to establish who people have worked with ... and what their actual cred / reputation is. Ask to meet them ... in person or via Skype and have your questions ready. Take notes. And be wary of clumsy / skillful attempts to "upsell" you. Trained coaches have a history of neglecting to mention that they were getting a cut from the ... "absolutely perfect (and pricey) course for you!!" ... that they pitching ["coaching"] you on. Caveat emptor.

OM coaching trainees have been known to offer – unsolicited – their [often] clumsy training advice. If you discover that any coach 'trainees' (or actual trained OM coaches for that matter) will be present during an OM / OM Circle ... check in with your partner and get on the same page about whether you are a request for coaching *during that OM only.* And then inform the coach / observer ahead of time.

The standard practice of OM coaches – both official and 'unofficial' coaches – was (until recently) to do live OM coaching wherever possible. In 90 seconds of live OM coaching ... by a knowledgable OMer / coach ... a lot of little mistakes and wrong turns can be gently observed, identified, and corrected. This remains the gold standard for how to be trained in how to OM.

Sharing the Practice: this is about how you talk others about your OM practice. The concepts of 'right range,' "I'm full," and 'consent' are useful here. (See entries for all 3 terms.)

A Guide to Somatic OMing

Keep in mind OM is an edgy non-mainstream *sexual* activity.

New OMers – or people just curious and investigating OM – have to navigate a litany of questions and concerns (from themselves and others):

1. Is OM a cult?
2. What do I think about strangers touching a woman's pussy?
3. What do I think of women getting support … for having [their own] orgasms?
4. How do I talk about this … with my family / friends / colleagues / strangers?
5. What is responsible conduct … and what is "over the line"?
6. What *is* possible?

New OMers tend to be bubbly in their enthusiasm … but these are dangerous times. Think carefully before you speak. Just because your privacy is not at risk or not an issue for you (at present) … doesn't mean that of others won't be. And … in these uncertain times … women bear far more risk than men in these conversations. Don't unwittingly 'out' someone … who is not *actively* promoting their professional services (coaching, teaching) in this area.

"Sunshine makes the best disinfectant."

Encourage people to ask questions. Challenge rote answers and rote thinking. Pay attention to actual results. OM is amazing … for some people. And OM isn't for everyone.

"I'm Full:" there two different uses of "I'm Full" in OM. (See the entries for "Filling Up" and "Full.")

The first "I'm full" is when someone (usually women) has noticed that they have reached a saturation point in their OM practice. They no longer have a chronic low-level background hunger for limbic connection. They have reached a place of abundance, somatically. (This can normally take 2+ years of a steady OM practice.)

The second "I'm full" comes in conversation ... or in the course of listening to a lengthy explanation (say, about OM). Basically, there may come a point where "your ears are full" ... and even if they keep talking ... nothing more is going 'in.' Among [some] OMers ... we give ourselves permission to say, "I'm full." The courteous / prudent response is ... to stop talking immediately (if it is just the 2 of you). After all, the glazed look in their eyes usually confirms ... *nothing* more will go in. They need a break. If, however, the speaker chooses *not* to stop talking ... well, in OM we would call that "overstroking" – stroking past the point of pleasure. It is a newbie mistake.

It is explained in detail here ... https://www.facebook.com/theOMrepor...

"Let's Pause:" (... or just, "Pause.") This is an optional communication within the actual OM. Generally, (although rarely used) it is used by the strokee.

[Intellectual] Peacocking: this is a form of intellectual 'showmanship' ... used to attract the interest of potential partners ... and usually (although not always) performed by men. It occurs often with new men (and a few women) when they first come to OM. The excitement and titillation of stroking a woman's clitoris ... kicks in some of their habituated routines for getting 'noticed.'

People 'peacocking' tend to dominate the conversation they enter ... and indulge in lengthy over-intellectualizations. They are also prone to be competitive ... so dueling 'peacocks' generate a lot of traffic / words. An expensive downside around OM and OM conversations is ... women tend to become silent and wander off. Their voices tend to disappear. And the peacocks – since there is an "apparently" vibrant (and frequently male-dominated) conversation taking place – think everything is peachy.

The challenge comes in calling the peacocks out. Since they are comfortable and familiar with this form of 'dialogue' – and they earn social status 'points' (at least

A Guide to Somatic OMing

in the past) by showing "winning" displays of their "powers of communication" – they are *very* attached to staying on that field. They are not easily dislodged. People who peacock also tend to be disconnected from their bodies. (Hence, the expression "they are in their heads.")

If a person peacocking doesn't already have the concept of "peacocking" in their vocabulary ... it is almost impossible to introduce it *while* they are in that mode. They will jump at the chance to argue with you about it ... and they will likely see this as yet another opportunity for peacocking! It is best to withdraw and bring it up when someone else – who can be observed – is peacocking. Experienced OMers (who have this distinction) ... when called out for 'peacocking' ... will stop immediately and check in with their body to see if that is accurate. There is a noticeable somatic address ('feeling') ... that often shows up in a guy's body when he is 'peacocking' ... kind of a high-pitched energetic buzzing. It is very noticeable once you become aware of it. The smart ones simply say, "got it" ... and, well ... stop talking. And reconnect.

Once people [men] put in enough time in the nest, their need to talk about it changes. They can listen more.

The valued currency in OM culture ... is conversations with people deeply connected to their bodies ... who display – and show support for – authentic, truthful, vulnerable communications ... and that show awareness and sensitivity for people's fluid 'right ranges' – and consent / agency.

* * *

:: The Basic Practice ::

The practice of [Classic] OM, at its simplest, consists of the following steps:

- asking for an OM
- setting up a nest and supplies
- getting in position
- pre-OM grounding
- noticing step
- gloving up
- safeport … first contact
- starting the OM / starting the timer
- the Lube Stroke
- more stroking
- 2-minute warning
- downstrokes
- the OM is ended / time is called
- pelvic grounding
- towel step
- additional post-OM grounding as needed
- frames exchanged
- the nest is put away
- the OM is complete.

A Guide to Somatic OMing

OM Jargon

The following are some instances of relevant OM jargon or slang.

A[n OM] Practice

OM is a practice, like Tai Chi or yoga. It is not for everyone. As a practice, its effects are cumulative. The more you do, the more you learn. Like Tai Chi and yoga … OM has its own somatic landscape … its own common terrain. Practitioners around the globe may encounter strikingly similar somatic experiences – without ever hearing either about other people's experience or of that particular type of experience. As in a 'landscape' … certain large landmarks will be experienced by most practitioners … if they practice long enough. And as in a 'landscape' … other features may be more local, more intimate … and be experienced by only a small number of practitioners. And having a long practice will not mean you will visit every possible area or somatic 'address' in the land of OM / orgasm. Just as we tend to be habitual as tourists, so too will we show up as OMers … unconsciously visiting the same places – or the same 'type' of places – over and over again. This landscape is the landscape of a woman in orgasm.

Since OM is a community-based practice, however, when we hear the reports of other 'travelers of OM' … we get a glimpse into what may lie off our beaten path.

A woman 'who has a gorgeous [OM] practice' … will have a vibrant and moist / hydrating relationship with her pussy, her sex, and her entire body. (This is not a 'goal' … just an address that may be visited.) She is less 'in charge' and more an equal 'ally' of her pussy. She is curious, adventuresome, courageous, and … sometimes 'still as a lake' … in her OMs. Her body knows the breadth of the 'landscape' … and she is completely at home there. A person who strokes women … will be always a guest in this domain … and if they are wise and skilled and patient … a gracious, supportive, and welcomed guest.

Asymmetric Practice: "OM is an asymmetric practice." This means that women's clitorises are stroked ... with no expectation of reciprocation. There no "owe-sies." In western cultures women have often been conditioned to push their sex down ... often hiding it or shaming it out of sight. The intent of OM is to create a safe space where women can attend to – and honor – their need for sexual engagement. OM is a space that supports women's empowerment around *their* sex and *their* voices.

The opposite of an asymmetric practice would be a symmetric practice, best represented by "commerce-based sex" ... where "I'll do you, if you do me." Women, for the most part, come out on the short end of such transactions. Hence, the creation of OM.

Goalless Practice: OM is described as a goalless practice. This means several things. First, it takes 'climax' or 'going over' off the table as a concrete objective ... dramatically reducing performance anxiety – for *both* partners. There is no *there* to get to ... no 'destination' to use as a cruel yardstick. OM is designed to give women as much unencumbered limbic connection as their bodies require – no strings attached. OM helps both partners ... in its function as a meditation ... tune in and get better at listening to their own bodies, as well as that of their partners.' This improvement happens naturally, over time. You just need to show up, be present, and do the practice.

Wax on, wax off.

Solid Practice: this a vague term. Generally, it will mean – for a woman – that she has cultivated a regular stroker or strokers, that she OMs regularly and on at least a weekly basis, that she has had at least 100 OMs, that she understands and consistently honors the [OM] container, that she gives clean frames consistently, that she is comfortable talking about her pussy and orgasm with other OMers (just women is fine), and she is able and comfortable asking questions as well as asking for help when she needs it. That is to say, she plugs into community well.

A Guide to Somatic OMing

For a stroker – particularly a male stroker – having a solid practice will mean (again, generally) ... that first off, they have a solid understanding of – and demonstrates consistent respect for – the OM Container, that they have OMed at least 100 times, that they OM regularly and at least a couple of times each week, that they gives clean frames consistently, that they are comfortable listening to women speak about their pussy and orgasm (without getting 'hooked' into thinking this is a prequel to a romance / courtship conversation), and they are able and comfortable asking questions as well as asking for help when they need it. That is to say, they plug into community well. Additionally, the more partners they have OMed with – and who recommend them – the more chance that they will be a solid stroker.

For both women and their strokers, the more OM partners they have over time – particularly experienced OM partners – the quicker they [tend to] learn and the wider their body of knowledge. The traveling analogy holds up well here. If you travel with the same person, you tend to visit the same type of places. If you instead spend time traveling with different partners, you tend (easily) to visit a much broader range of places and have a more diverse range of experiences.

Note for both married / monogamous strokees and strokers who choose to OM *only* with their partners ... the "has-OMed-with-many-others" will understandably be off the table. A 'solid practice' for them will look a little different, accordingly. A solid practice is still possible – and potentially deeply rewarding.

Being Stroked: [In an OM] this refers to one person strokes a woman's clit. [Outside of an OM] this can refer (metaphorically) to any delivered communication. We are said to "stroke" someone when we speak with them. Our communications will impact them ... much like an OM ... sending them up ... or grounding them ... sometimes "peaking" them (possibly triggering an emotionally numinous end result, such as laughter, crying, or another energetic release). When stroking someone – whether in an OM or in a conversation in 'normal' life – strive to be fully present and fully in your body.

A Guide to Somatic OMing

Starting the OM: this refers to the actual start of an OM ... the first stroke (which is the lube stroke). Everything prior is just prep ... getting into position, putting the gloves on, setting the timer. If you hear "they have started the OM" ... do not interrupt (or make noise). Wait out the completion of the OM ... which is 15 minutes + about 7 to 10 minutes for grounding / frames etc.

Ending the OM: Normally, the OM ends with a two-minute warning ("2 minutes") by the stroker to their partner, followed 2 minutes later by the stroker calling, "Time." At that point, slow downward pelvic compressions (grounding) may be administered, and maybe some thigh squeezes (depending on the woman's personal preferences), followed (depending on which variation a stroker learned – and what the woman actually prefers) by the towel stroke. The woman then finishes off toweling / pussy clean-up ... to her satisfaction. The two then exchange frames. The woman gets up ... and her partner starts putting away the nest. (Generally, the stroker assembles and disassembles the nest ... leaving the woman free to a) shift emotionally in prep for the OM, and b) continue feeling into her body, post-OM.) In cases where the nest doesn't need to be broken down right away, the woman may hang out and chill for a bit. Ask her what she wants you to do. No hugs. If *she* wants to hug, do it later ... at least 15 minutes post-OM. Hugs screw up the energy of the nest ... and while *she* may like it in the moment, her body / pussy will be pissed. Keep a clean container. (And if *you* – her stroker – want a hug, walk it off. Hugs are great ... but they don't belong around a nest / in an OM.)

Oh ... and under *no* circumstances (the latest version [1.2.2] of OM Container doc is incorrect here) should you skip safeporting her if you need to step over a woman who is lying in a nest. Even if she says she is "fine" ... her body / pussy will tense up. And remember.

Wrap Up the OM: once "Time!" is called ... the following steps remain: pelvic grounding, the towel stroke, more grounding, take off the gloves, exchange frames, tidy / pack up the nest. This is "wrapping up the OM."

A Guide to Somatic OMing

Significant Markers

Uninterrupted: the OM should be uninterrupted. The woman is lying on her back with her pussy exposed. It is a very vulnerable position. No traffic. No visitors. No guests. No surprises.

Turn the smartphones to silent (not just to vibrate). No alarms, no 'notifications,' no text messages, no phone calls, no "vibrating" alerts. (Take the time ... before an actual OM ... to figure out how to best switch your phone to "OM Mode" – and off "OM Mode" again later.)

After the nest is put away ... turn your smartphones and notifications back on.

Getting in Position: this refers to the OM positions for the woman and her stroker.

The woman lays down in the OM nest ... with her pants (or skirt) and panties *only* removed ... her pussy visible and positioned directly over the OM towel ... and her knees bent and her legs 'butterflied" open ... and her knees supported by cushions / pillows on either side. Her head is supported by a pillow (unless she prefers to lie flat.)

Her stroker carefully positions themselves on the woman's right side ... so that the stroker's left leg is over the woman's belly ... left knee bent and the left foot supported by additional cushions if need be (so that the stroker's left leg does not put pressure on the woman's midsection) ... and the stroker's right leg is bent at the knee ... and lying on (or close to) the floor ... and underneath (and supporting) the woman's butterflied (bent) right leg. If the stroker is small relative to the woman, additional firm pillows or cushions may be required to raise their butt up far enough that the stroker's left leg clears (doesn't put pressure on) the woman's midsection.

A Guide to Somatic OMing

Generally, the stroker's OM supplies – lube jar, gloves, & timer – are to the stroker's left ... within easy reach. (The gloves should be on something sanitary. Some strokers place the gloves on the OM towel. Others use a second – clean – OM towel for staging.)

OM Towel: this is placed under a woman's pussy ... usually placed in its approximate location before the OM partners take their position ... and adjusted after the woman lies down (with appropriate safeporting).

OM towels are very often clean washcloths or small hand towels ... specifically reserved for OMing (and touching a woman's pussy). They should be soft and preferably all natural. It isn't necessary that they be white – just very clean and hygienic.

A larger towel (even full size) may be used in cases where 1) a woman is on her period and may have a heavy flow, or 2) a woman has discovered that she occasionally squirts in her OM. (For more on OM Towels click here.)

Timer: this is a small digital clock or smartphone app ... which the stroker – or a timekeeper in group OMs (OM circles) – uses to keep time in the OM. Timekeepers in OM circles are responsible for saying (once everyone is ready), "Begin," ... at the start of the OM ... and giving the 2-minute (to completion) warning ... and the final, "Time!" ... at the end of the OM.

Noticing (formerly Obnosing): this a key early step in the basic OM. It is the act – by the stroker – of describing ... in purely value-neutral sensory terms ... the stroke's pussy. 'Value-neutral' means avoiding any kind of 'judging' language ... for instance, "beautiful," "stunning," "gorgeous," etc. are all judgements / evaluations by the observer. Judging language *has* to be evaluated by the listener (stroker) ... "do they really mean it?" ... "they used more flattering language last time" ... "I think he just wants to sleep with me" – in other words, head-tripping. OM is designed to leave all of that social jockeying behind ... and get *both* parties out of their heads ... and into their bodies.

A Guide to Somatic OMing

So instead, the stroker is limited to words that are factually and observably true and accurate (colors, shadows, shapes, textures, etc.).

This is a ritual communication ... which helps the woman lovingly reconnect with – and bring approval to – her sex. It also helps the stroker connect to the woman in front of him ... as a real flesh-and-blood person ... and not as an abstract 'entity' that they will be stroking momentarily. All genders in the west may have unconsciously – or even consciously – stigmatized the sex organs in general ... and those of women in particular. Women have been taught by western society for millennia ... that women's sex organs are 'filthy,' unclean, forbidden, an embarrassment, dangerous, taboo, and even disgusting.

The act of hearing her pussy ... described (with an air of approval and acceptance) with words – that by their very nature – bring her pussy into the light ... is immensely healing and frequently deeply moving for many women.

Note that a variation of this action can be done alone by women with mirrors ... and can also help them reconnect with – and bring approval to – their sex. (A slightly longer version of semi-public 'Noticing' has been done in OM-related classes exclusively for women. In these old classes (2007) ... women offered the same neutral descriptions of each others' pussies ... slowly ... one at a time. Again ... restoring social and personal approval to women's sex / pussies.)

Note also that many practitioners who OM often and regularly together ... habitually drop this step (at the strokee's request only, of course) ... with their regular partners. I would suggest to those women that they consider revisiting the Noticing Step "every 5th OM" (or something similar) – and definitely put it in for new strokers / partners. It helps the strokers connect too.

And Pussy likes thoughtful attention.

Obnosing: this is an outdated term still used by older strokers ... that has been replaced in recent years by the term 'noticing' and 'the noticing step.' (See the term "noticing" above.)

A Guide to Somatic OMing

Gloves: OM strokers use gloves when they stroke their partners' clits. There are 3 basic glove materials: latex, nitrile, or vinyl. Some women have an allergy to a specific material. Since the gloves are used to prevent bacteria or diseases from being introduced to the pussy (or to the stroker), there are some hygiene practices and tips to be aware of. This post has a detailed rundown on the topic of OM gloves: https://www.facebook.com/theOMreport/posts/800109966743410

Lube: lube is an integral part of OMing. At the start – and indeed duration – of most OMs, most women lack sufficient natural pussy lubrication to stroke her clit without causing discomfort and / or irritation. A lube is required. The requirements for a good OM lube are fairly narrow … it needs to not dissipate or evaporate before the end of the 15-minute session and to maintain its viscosity and slipperiness over that same period. And – most importantly – it mustn't trigger any allergic reactions or irritate the woman's pussy in any way.

A custom lube recipe was refined by the Warehouse residents during 2006 – 07, eventually being packaged and sold as "OneStroke" Lube. This the lube most commonly used in OMing. The main ingredients were all organic, and included beeswax, shea butter, beeswax, and grapefruit seed extract.

(See also **Lube Alternatives,** below, and here for more on Lube in general.)

Lube Alternatives: OneStroke Lube (produced and recommended by OT and most used by veteran OMers), coconut oil, Honey Girl Personal Lubricant from Hawaii, Albolene (primary ingredient is mineral oil), Egyptian Magic, the Australian OMers seem to like Brauer Papaw.

UTIs: this stands for Urinary Tract Infection. This is a pain for women and generally requires them to take a break from OMing. OMs – done right – are extremely sanitary and safe.

However, if a stroker is careless … they can contaminate the lube or get contaminants on the gloves. Watch what the gloves touch. Have an extra pair handy … in case you need to change your position (and by shifting your weight

– end up inadvertently leaning on your gloved hands). Watch your lube handling. (For more on Lube Handling see here.)

Peaking: this is changing the direction of the stroke before the sensation starts to drop off. It is applicable in OMs and in ordinary interactions. (See the entry "peak(s).")

2-Minute Warning: an OM is 15 minutes long. At the 13-minute mark, the stroker (or the timekeeper in group OMs) announces clearly (yet not *too* loudly) "2 Minutes" … to let the strokee(s) know that the OM will end in 2 minutes. Both the strokee and the stroker … should begin lowering the energy in the OM … in preparation for the OM ending and subsequent grounding.

The stroker wants to avoid leaving the strokee hung out on a peak at the end of the OM. However, it is a practice … so if she is 'hanging' … that is fine … end the OM promptly on time. Keep the container. One of the things her pussy will be evaluating … is whether the stroker can be counted on to keep their agreements.

(Note: a sneaky tactic of OM container "poachers" is … they will attempt to *raise* the women's energy … in the last 2 minutes of the OM … in order to 'get her' to break the container … and ask for "just a couple of minutes more." Strokers should be bringing you down in the last 2 minutes. Do not put up with container 'poaching.')

Two minutes. Wind it down people.

"Time!": this is what is called out at the end of an OM. An OM is 15 minutes in length. At the 13-minute mark, the stroker (or a timekeeper if it is a group OM) calls *"2 minutes"* … followed 2 minutes later by *"Time!"* In both cases … the announcements should clear and just loud enough to be heard clearly. Shouting isn't [usually] necessary.

Grounding: this a core distinction of OM. It mirrors the use of "grounding" electrical current. Basically, in an OM the woman (strokee) may experience heightened states of arousal for a sustained period of time (15 minutes). "Grounding" here refers to an assortment of physical techniques to "bring the strokee's energy down" – safely. The strokee – if left in a significantly elevated state (aka, "high") – may fail to perform basic manual tasks safely like drive safely, use knives in a kitchen, or cross a crosswalk safely. The bulk of their attention – if they are not grounded sufficiently – will still be focused on the lingering internal (pleasurable) sensations.

The primary technique a stroker uses at the conclusion of the OM … is a firm pressure down and towards the strokee's head (basically a 45° angle) by the stroker's open palm … placed over the woman's pubic bone. [exact directions can be found <u>here</u> in the OM Container PDF]. (Some women can take – and want – *a lot* of pressure on their pubic bone. Proceed cautiously … and check-in with your partner – often.) Other techniques include pressing down on the strokee's inner thighs … or even – after the OM is over – (and at the request of the strokee) standing face-to-face … and *gently* stepping stepping on the front of the strokee's feet (no more than 3 inches of overlap).

All of these techniques are likely to "bring the strokee down" … help them 'get back in their body.' Women often describe being grounded as a sensation of energy flooding out of their body … with a feeling similar to 'letting the air out of a balloon.'

After the OM, the energy [in her body] will 'want' to come down. The trick is to find pleasurable, non-disruptive ways to do this "coming down." Other actions that can be used (post-OM) … are doing gardening or cleaning, doing aikido or hot yoga, soaking in a hot bath, getting a massage, or even certain kinds of sex. All of these can help a person "get back in their body." If a person is not sufficiently grounded … they may unconsciously elect to "finish" coming down … by arguing with someone or picking a fight – both great (although disruptive) ways to clear a lot of energy fast out of the body. Keep in mind OM is designed to assist the woman in building up and being able to *hold* ever-increasing amounts of energy in their body. Grounding makes sure those build-ups of energy are sufficiently dissipated … so that the woman can go about her

A Guide to Somatic OMing

day, post-OM, and be productive and efficient if necessary.

Note that strokers can experience their own highs ... which may require grounding. They should handle their own grounding themselves, as a rule. Push-ups, crunches, or Tai Chi are some additional options. I'll say this again ... strokers should tend – and tend well – to their own grounding. The last thing that a woman wants to hear post-OM ... is that she "needs" to look after their stroker's needs. Generally, the woman's 'highs' are much richer and get much more complex. Part of a stroker's job ... is to close up the container after the OM. This means leaving the woman in good shape ... and sufficiently grounded to move on with her day. (Note that the stroker is *assisting* the strokee ... in meeting her needs – when she says, "enough" – stop.)

Historically, the developers of OM pushed hard on finding out how little grounding was needed – and how little they could get away with. OM Circles can be an example of this. Not all women, after every OM ... can get by with 2 minutes of grounding (typical in some OM Circles). Some women, after some OMs ... need *much* more grounding. As much as half an hour of additional grounding on some occasions (for some women) is necessary. Not makeouts, grounding. Not flirting, grounding. Strokers ... if you are grounding them ... the OM is still taking place – keep the OM Container and keep it clean. Women ... as you learn more about your bodies ... adjust your OM requests and safeport your OM partners. ("I may need about 20 minutes of additional grounding when we OM on Tuesday. I may not ... but ... does that work for you?")

Strokees and strokers ... keep an OM journal. Make notes about what works, what you have tried, ... and ask around for other OMer's grounding tips.

Grounding is an essential form of self-care. We don't just deal with energy surges in OMs. They can happen when we get great / awful news ... experience a physical or emotional jolt ... or finish a marathon task. Become more conscious of the energy shifts in your body ... and when you need to come down ... find a way to do so – ground yourself – pleasurably.

A Guide to Somatic OMing

Towel Stroke: the towel stroke is the end of the physical part of the OM ... and is intended to remove excess lube and fluids from the pussy. (Removal of the gloves and the exchange of frames follows shortly afterwards.) **Note whether the fabric of the towel is baby-soft (good) ... or harsh and abrasive (bad). Safeport your strokee and ask what she would like for the towel stroke – for you to do it, or does she want to do it.** (For more on the Towel see here.)

Different versions of how to do the Towel Stroke exist. When OMing with a new partner, ask ahead of the OM what Towel Stroke method they know about. Defer to what the strokee prefers.

Sharing Frames: this a step at the very conclusion of the OM. Both practitioners ... exchange 2 sensory-specific frames each ... from moments in the OM when they felt a specific pleasurable / interesting / annoying sensation.

The design of this step is ... to support creating bridges based on sensation ... first between your body and you ability to language *what* you feel – cleanly. And the second bridge ... is with another person – in this case, your OM partner. By sharing sensation reports ('frames') from *your* experience of the same OM ... your body is able to "check in" with the other person's body. It is not uncommon for partners to focus on the same moments ... and use the same language.

Our bodies are already talking to each other during the OM ... exchanging and shaping and reshaping energy. The frames step gives them a chance to check in. And we learn a little bit more. (See the entries on "Frames" and "Clean Frames.")

* * *

:: The Pussy / Anatomy ::

Pussy

Part of [Classic] OM training ... is to recover a place of honor in language ... for women's sex. Their pussies / cunts / vaginas have *literally* been called ... "unmentionables." The use of clinical language (e.g., "vagina" or "genitals") ... and euphemisms (e.g., "down there" or "the nether regions") ... were both considered ways to create "distance" ... from the "dangerous & unseemly subject matter."

So ... the creator of OM (a woman) settled on 'pussy' as a female-centric, sex-positive term ... that women – and their allies – could celebrate ... with their voices. 'Pussy' is not the only acceptable term ... it is merely a starting point, a shared cultural gateway for OMers ... to bring approval to a woman's sex – and its expression, orgasm, in the world.

In the early stages of a woman's OM training during the Warehouse Days ... she was encouraged to actually look at her pussy – in the presence of other women in her class. And bring her approval to her pussy. And she was encouraged ... gently ... to set aside vague and concealing euphemisms ... in favor of saying – loud and proud – 'pussy' when referring to her own ... or other women's sex.

The point wasn't to replace her language.

It was to reclaim her voice ... and – publicly – associate honor and magnificence with her sex. She was free to develop her own preferences, her own language.

Use of the word 'pussy' is merely an exercise, a custom. And its use is maintained in contemporary OM culture as a reminder to veterans – and also as training support for new OMers.

Clit (Clitoris): the clit is located in a woman's pussy, near the top, this is a small round area of tissue and what the stroker actually strokes. (Technically what stroker actually strokes is just the one o'clock position on the exposed tip of the clit – with the one o'clock position being *from the woman's perspective.*) It is [usually] partially covered by the clitoral hood. Clits vary *greatly* in sizes. Upon a woman becoming aroused, her clit *may* swell (become engorged with blood) greatly. In some women their engorged clit looks like a small penis … and actually protrudes from the surrounding tissue. Some clits are tiny … and remain covered in tissue even during arousal.

Generally, at the start of an OM the stroker may have some trouble finding – and staying on – the clit with their stroking finger. That's okay. OM is a practice.

Gradually, during the OM … as the woman's arousal increases … the clit swells and protrudes somewhat.

Strokers note … *never* make a woman wrong for the size of her clit – or any other features her pussy (or body). This is where you "bring your approval" – no matter what you encounter. *She is perfect.* Work with what is there. Do the best you can. Study what's there, learn, and adapt.

Remember: stroking a woman is a privilege.

Wikipedia :: https://en.wikipedia.org/wiki/Clitoris

A Guide to Somatic OMing

[Clitoral] Hood: the clitoral hood is the fold of skin that surrounds and protects the glans (top) of the clitoris. It also covers the external shaft of the clitoris. In OM the stroker *gently* uses the edge of their gloved left thumb to pull back the hood so they can stroke the *very* top of the clitoris – specifically the upper left hand quadrant of the woman's clit.

In some women in a high state of arousal, their clit protrudes from their hood a lot very quickly … or is normally quite large (like a small penis). In other women, their clit can be tiny in size … even when they are aroused. In some cases, the hood can be difficult to find and to keep retracted. It will take practice. (See Wikipedia.)****

1 O'Clock Position: this is a location on the woman's clitoris (the orientation of the imagined clock … is from the viewpoint of the woman, not her stroker). Rather than a vague instruction … "just stroke her clit" … the instruction to "stroke the one o'clock position on her clit" … serves to train the stroker to adjust their perception … with an eye to making very minuscule adjustments. Over time, strokers learn to perceive the tip of the clit … as a vast terrain.

Introitus: this is the entrance to the entrance to the pussy. (See wikipedia.) In a [Classic] OM, the gloved right thumb (*tip only*) is placed at the very bottom of the introitus / pussy entrance … to help ground the strokee during the OM.

Inner Lips: these are also called the labia minora. (See wikipedia.) The clit and clitoral hood are located above where the inner lips meet at the top. With some women, the lips must – carefully – be moved aside / opened in order to actually stroke the clit.

Outer Lips: these are also called the labia majora. (See wikipedia.) The clit and clitoral hood are located above where the outer lips meet at the top. With some women, the lips must – carefully – be moved aside / opened in order to actually stroke the clit.

* * *

:: Orgasm ::

Orgasm

In OM 'orgasm' is defined in a unique, nontraditional way. It works. Whereas orgasm is traditionally associated with the distinctly male act of climax / ejaculation ... in OM, orgasm is taken to be the whole of the wave ... that precedes ... and includes ... and follows ... 'climax.'

In the culture of OM, orgasm is energy ... and all [somatic] energy is orgasmic. Access and openness to [a woman in] orgasm ... is the medium through which an OM practitioner reconnects to their body and restores a more natural dialogue with their intuitions, intuitive self, and their own deeper wisdom. (For a more detailed explanation of OM's model of orgasm, please see Nicole Daedone's (the founder of OM) book, 'Slow Sex.')

   [a] **Woman in Orgasm:** this is the central focus of OM. It is not just that OM was designed to source and support women's empowerment around their sex and their voice. Women's orgasms have proven to be a lush source of energy, discovery, and exotic altered states ... over the years. Men's orgasm [usually] pales when placed in comparison.

   Contraction: [in an OM] the pussy may physically contract, which can be detected by the stroker as the pussy closes [sometimes repeatedly] on the stroker's thumb tip as it rests on the bottom of the entrance to the woman's introitus.

More generally, a contraction is a withdrawal or diminishment of the energy [in a person]. A person bursting into laughter can be said to be expanding [energetically] ... while if they stop suddenly when a teacher enters the room, they can be said to be contracting [energetically]. Energy – whether in a room, an individual, or an OM – ebbs and flows constantly. It rarely stays att the same level in nature. The 'ebbs' are contractions, the 'flows' are expansions.

Going Over: OM uses an expanded redefinition of orgasm. Within OM's model of orgasm, traditional climax is simply one part of much richer tableau. OMers, however, rarely say 'climax.' Instead, the experience we call 'climax' … is called 'going over.' Use of the phrase 'going over' deintensifies the report … and creates space – and support – for the expanded orgasm model.

Every time a woman "goes over" (climaxes) in an OM, her energy drops and she has to start over. It is a lot like surfing. I can paddle a short way out … catch a small wave … ride it for a few seconds. And then my ride is over. And I have to paddle back out. Or I paddle for a longer time … catch a big wave … and have a *much* longer ride. Climax is equivalent to the wipeout at the end of riding the wave.

The more experienced women OMers figure this out – whether they have been taught this or not. They discover they like "riding the wave of orgasm" during an OM. And when they climax / go over … they find they have to start over (paddle back out) … building up energy. The sweet spot … is riding the wave – and just like surfers – to avoid wiping out as long as they can. Experienced women – and some newbies – can start an OM already in high state of turn-on / orgasm (their pussy may already be having contractions) … and they just intensify that orgasm throughout the OM … and ride that ever-increasing wave of orgasm – without going over – for the *whole OM.*

In the start of a woman's OM practice, they may be "hungry" for going over / climax. The coaching women were given during the Warehouse years was … to have "going over' be the focus of their "research" (a phase of focused exploration on one particular aspect of OM or one's turn-on). Eventually, they would become sated … and bored / curious. And their practice would move on to a broader vision: exploring their own orgasm.

So in OM, the point [for experienced OMers] isn't "going over" (climax). It is to ride the wave *just* inside the edge ... of going over ... in a state of heightened sensation ... for as long as they can.

That is called "the ride."

Getting Off: this a rich complex OM term. Very broadly, it refers to a state of openness that allows the energy to flow easily. More narrowly, it can refer to a person permitting themselves ... to be aroused, turned-on, or otherwise energetically engaged in a pleasurable way. The antithesis may be a deliberate (conscious or unconscious) tightening or tensing ... or a numbing of sensation ... or a dialing back in sensation. OM is designed to provide a safe space for a woman to 'get off' ... and to explore what that means to her.

Peak(s): an important part of OM is the concept of orgasm and waves. When stroking a woman ... for a while it may feel like we are going "up" ... and then a shift in her energy [orgasm] will occur ... and we will be going "down" energetically ... until another shift occurs – and we are going "up" again. The stroker's job is to follow and anticipate the shifts in energy ... and ... a second before it fades ... change the direction ... with our stroke. This preserves and maximizes energetic 'momentum.'

The apex or top of these waves are called 'peaks.'

Outside of OM, we use to the metaphor of 'peaks' to refer to energetic 'peaks' in our daily interactions / conversations. When a friend tells a funny story ... the "punchline" (when it is skillfully delivered) ... is the 'peak' of the story – and the experience. There may be a wave of laughter and applause immediately afterwards ... and then the energy dissipates. Until someone builds it back up ... with another story / conversation / communication. OMing sensitizes us to the ebb and flow of energy ... in ordinary interactions – and allows us to better maximize, utilize, and harvest naturally occurring 'peaks.' It has the potential to make us better communicators, better leaders, ... and better listeners.

A Guide to Somatic OMing

It also makes leaving a party more memorable when you leave on a peak … rather than when all of the "juice" (energy) is sucked out of it.

Engorged Lips: one of the visible signs of arousal (turn-on) is the engorgement of the woman's pussy lips. When engorged … they often swell in size and can become redder in color.

Strokers are advised to keep their eyes on their partners' pussies. The physiological changes they undergo give real-time limbic feedback as to the state of the woman's arousal … and hence, the state of the OM.

Squirting: "Squirting" is when a woman ejaculates ("squirts") a clear liquid out of her pussy … when she is in a state of high arousal. It is not pee. It can squirt quite far … in a few women. (Short article On Female Ejaculation / "Squirting.")

This can happen occasionally (or regularly, with some women) and handling it should not be treated as a "big deal." It is considered part of the Sacred Messy. It should be supported gracefully (a larger towel may be needed) and 'clean approval' placed on the strokee (some women have shame or embarrassment around squirting). Some women are enamored of their squirting – support that. It's their pussy … whatever they choose to celebrate about it should be supported.

Women: please safeport your partners around any tendencies to squirt and how you would like to best be supported around that.

Strokers: create a space of low-key approval and acceptance for your partner. (If squirting happens … cool. If not … cool. Avoid making it an OM 'goal.')

* * *

:: Community ::

ROLES

OMer: this is a person who OMs ... i.e., practices Orgasmic Meditation.

Strokee: in OM, a strokee is the person being stroked, and is always a woman. What is being stroked is the woman's clitoris ... by the stroker's left-hand index fingertip.

Stroker: in OM, a stroker is the person stroking the woman. A stroker can be any gender, although it is most often a man in most communities. What is being stroked is the woman's clitoris ... by the stroker's left-hand index fingertip.

Veteran OMer: this is an experienced OMer. They should be able to handle training and supporting a new OMer.

(See also the terms "Senior Women," above ... and "Veteran Stroker," below.)

Senior Women: this refers to experienced women OMers. In the past, this often meant women who had assisted in OM training repeatedly. They know (knew) the practice deeply ... on a formal and more importantly ... personal level. They had in excess of 750 OMs completed. They were founts of wisdom and guidance for new women ... and new men ... starting out in OM. During the Warehouse years (and prior) ... only women could teach OM and OM courses. So 'Senior Women' were much more valuable from a knowledge and leadership vantage point ... than 'Senior Men.' (In fact, experienced men weren't called 'Senior Men.' They were called 'veteran strokers.')

Veteran Stroker: this is a stroker who has accumulated experience stroking. They generally have at least 500 OMs and have OMed with five or more women – and have three or more strong recommendations. They hold the container well

A Guide to Somatic OMing

… and are not knocked off balance easily. They can handle a decent amount of energy well. They know the OM Container and OM & nest etiquette well.

Trained OMer: an OMer is a "trained" OMer if they have completed an in-person "How to OM" course … and / or received *thorough* OM coaching from an *experienced* coach or OMer. They should know the OM Model, the Container, and basic OM & nest etiquette.

It is recommended that … before OMing with any new partners … you ask about their training 'pedigree.' Since the length, structure, and content of OM courses have varied over time … it is important to get on the same page … with expectations about how an OM should go.

Ask for what specific OM training they have had, when, and who led it / taught it. Different teachers / coaches have different strengths. Ask them to walk you through what they understand an OM to consist of (stepwise). Compare notes with what you have learned. Ask them when they had their first OM … and how [roughly] many OMs they have completed. If they have less than 100, consider them a newbie … and expect that they may need some adjustments / support … around the basics.

If you are a woman … do not accept any pushback or gaslighting for asking these questions. It is your pussy. Screening and vetting are important safety steps. If something is unclear / hinky … check established online OM communities … and ask for clarification (use no names) from more experienced OMers.

Newbie OMer: this is a term for a new OMer. They typically require more attention, structure, patience, and support from their partners. Remember … everyone starts as a beginner.

If they are a stroker … they may have difficulty keeping track of OM protocols and sensations. They may need more frequent adjustments / requests … than more seasoned OMers. Particularly if they are men … they may have difficulty for a long while in actually feeling, and then distinguishing and naming /

languaging ... value-neutral sensations in their bodies ... for the exchange of frames at the completion of OMing.

If they are a strokee ... they may start with a heightened sense of vigilance / concern. They may forget to ask for what they want ... or ask in an awkward, indirect way. They may be disconnected from their pussies ... or have a deep sense of shame around their sex.

When you OM with a newbie ... remember that you are training them for future OM partners. Mind the container ... be gentle, kind, and consistent in your feedback. Help them deepen into their practice ... and connect cleanly to their own body.

OM Partners: this refers to the people one OMs with. OM partners may be one-offs: you may OM once and never again (a traveling OMer, for instance). Or they could be regular ("we OM every Tuesday night") or semi-regular partners. Every partner is different ... and provides a different experience of the landscape of orgasm. And every OM is unique. In general, the more OM partners you experience, the more you learn about OM, your body, and people.

Observer / Witness: in some [old] OM classes and some current OM Circles ... a practicing trained OMer may (for a variety of reasons) ... 'observe' an OM.

Sometimes in an OM Circle ... one person may be short a partner for one of the OM rounds. Depending on the group ... the custom may be that they have to wait outside the room until that OM round is complete. Or the custom may be ... they can just chill off to the side of the room ... soaking in the sights and sounds of the simultaneous OMs in the room (*highly* recommended!). Or they may be able to sit in and observe an experienced OM couple. (Generally, you should only ask to sit in and observe seasoned OMers ... in an OM Circle.)

In a class context, an observer may either be *more* experienced than the couple ... or less experienced. If more experienced, the observer may have been requested by the OMing couple ... to 'sit in' and observe ... with the idea to receive advice and / or observations from the observer later. (In special circumstances, the observer may be invited – before the start of the OM – by *both* partners to do live coaching during the OM. In this case ... the 'observer' ... is more accurately called a 'coach.' Coaching is just a role. Not all 'coaches' are paid. Some are just respected OMers with more experience OMing then the OM couple.

The Observer (sometimes called the witness) must have the explicit OK of the woman who's OM is being observed. Before the OM starts, the guest observer stages themselves ... near the nest, and in accord with the woman's (strokee's) preferences (she may find certain locations ... such as opposite her pussy ... unnerving or reassuring). The observer *may or may not* have a line of sight to the pussy. The observer ... once the OM starts ... should be still as a mouse – no gasps, no fidgeting, no questions, no exclamations. Just be quiet ... and observe. They might do so with their eyes open ... or they might shut their eyes in order to better feel the shifts in energy. After they OM is over ... the observer *may* be invited to share frames. Do so graciously. Avoid bubbling or chattering. You are a guest ... to a very intimate act. After the OM is fully wrapped up ... check in with the OM partners ... to see if a deeper conversation / sharing of notes is appropriate. Any details of the OM should be held in the strictest confidence – including especially who you observed.

All of that said, I would recommend more OMers 'sit in' on [experienced] OMers more often. OMers can get a bit greedy about getting their OMs in ... and yet ... observing another couple's OMs ... can be an eye-opening experience. People who have done so ... have reported picking up things that they had forgotten, getting insights into their own practice, and gaining a multilevel deepening appreciation for the practice. (As a rule, however ... avoid sitting in on a spouse's OM with another stroker ... until both of your practices are rock solid. The experience can deeply vulnerable, unsettling, revealing, and / or triggering to one or both spouses. Avoid the drama. Learn from strangers and friends and actual coaches.)

Practice Holder [for a Community]: when the Warehouse Community was around, Nicole led the women – and the community overall. But she had a highly trained and skilled [male] partner, J, who functioned as the "Practice Holder" for the community. His job was to take the temperature of the community – and particularly the men – and see whether it was expanding or contracting, where the men were at energetically ... and basically see what adjustments might be needed ... to enable the group to continue to thrive while fulfilling its mission.* He counseled Nicole and she listened. (*The Warehouse Community's stated mission was to be 'messengers of orgasm' ... bringing OM out into the world.)

If a community was an OM, the community's practice holder ... keeps an eye on the community's container ... inside of its declared mission ... and makes – or recommends – adjustments to keep them on course.

Circle Holder: it is customary for some OMers to gather at one location and do simultaneous OMs (a "group" OM) ... in an "OM Circle." (And some OMers never attend an OM Circle, and may simply do private OMs only.) The circle holder is the one person charged with (or who volunteers) holding the integrity of the OM space for the duration of OMs (that means nest set-up, OMs, and the post-OM wrap up and stowing of the nests). This isn't some ethereal task. It is *very* practical. It means that person (the circle holder) watches for ... and heads off ... potential interruptions / disruptions ... like people knocking at the door, phones ringing, or other unwanted instances of the outside world pushing into the space. They will handle disturbances that arise ... so everyone else – in particular the women who are naked from the waist down – can relax and focus on the OM. Sometimes ... in large groups or high traffic ares ... this may mean the circle holder doesn't participate in the OMs. (They usually book private OMs later ... or get filled up some other time.) Other times, in smaller groups ... they may OM with the others ... *with* the understanding that if noises occur that warrant attention ... they will interrupt their OM and handle business. This prevents the situation from arising ... where a door is knocked on unexpectedly ... and *everyone* freezes ... while waiting to see *who* will finally get up and deal with it. (If they will participate in the group OMs, the circle holder is *always* a stroker – never a strokee. If they will *not* be participating in the group OMs, the circle holder can be any gender.) You want

A Guide to Somatic OMing

to avoid the situation where someone – known or unknown – enters the space without warning. This is why OM circles start on time. Part of the job of a circle holder will be to make sure that latecomers don't barge into the OM. They are part guard dog. And whatever they handle … they handle *quietly.* They can fill the others in later. Safe space to open … remember?

Community Holders: this is closely related to *circle holders* (see above). An OM community may be online (like the excellent Facebook OM Wiki Group) or local (a group of OMers know each other in parts of Los Angeles, for example). Unless the group is ad hoc and totally informal … it will have some structure, some history, and leaders. A 'community holder' is less explicit than a circle holder. It is someone who knows, understands, and cares about the practice of OM. They work to keep the local group of OMers (the "community) active, informed, and safe. They watch out for things that can disrupt or damage the community and / or its practice … like predatory males, a sloppy or inexperienced coach, predatory sales patterns, or internal disputes about the practice. They may act from time to time – or regularly – as teachers, coaches, facilitators, bomb defusers, gatekeepers, vetting agents, babysitters (literal or figurative), or [online] 'bouncers.' They need to have solid people skills, a calm and steady personality, a strong character and ethical foundation, and a willingness to *not* be in the spotlight. Good community holders often make great OM partners. 'Holding' a community … is a lot like OMing.

If there is not an organized OM community in your area, but you have a lot of local OMers … it usually means no one has stepped forward to be (or survived being) a community holder.* It tends to take a lot skill, a lot of flexibility, a lot of patience, a lot of time, a lot of energy, and a lot of bandwidth.

Timekeeper: in group OMs, one person is the timekeeper. They are responsible for saying (once everyone is ready), *"Begin,"* … at the start of the OM … and giving the 2-minute (to completion) warning … and the final, *"Time!"* … at the end of the OM. They may use a personal timer … or … if they are experienced … just use a clock within their line of sight. The announcements should clear and just loud enough to be heard clearly. Shouting shouldn't be necessary.

Projection is.

SCREENING

Vetting Partners: this is a vital part of establishing one's OM practice. You want first and foremost ... partners that you will be safe practicing with. You want partners who will hold the container well ... and not force you to shore up their leaky efforts. You want partners you can learn from – and with. And – this is important – partners whose energy your body finds nourishing.

And since OM is *not* a shortcut to dating or hooking up ... "attraction" or "types" can be set aside. Turn-on, energetic rapport, and integrity become the most important criteria in picking good OM partners.

And a big tip ... older OMers and OMers who do not fit the "Hollywood" aesthetic (young trim, a certain "look," a certain "size" ...) ... will often have more turn-on in their OMs – and more range – straight out the gate ... than the young folk. (See the entry for "Getting References" for more information on vetting partners.)

Lastly, in the current political climate you will want partners who can be discrete ... particularly online and in social media. Privacy, safety, and security are critical. It is in particular ... a dangerous time for women.

Screening Partners: this means to make sure that potential OM partners have a base level of skill and integrity ... as well as whatever personal requirements one may need.

Rep(utation) as an OMer: there two types of reps for OMers: that of a stroker and that of a strokee.

Given the precariousness of women's safety in the world today ... the stroker's rep / reputation is much more edgy. Do they hold a strong container? Are they an OM [Container] poacher? Are they coachable? Are they skilled in stroking, ... in grounding, ... in frames, ... in reading and stroking at the level of energy?

Are they polite / prompt / attentive / not clingy or needy? Do they show up smelly or dirty? Do they clip their nails wisely? Do they keep the lube uncontaminated and safe? Do they gaslight? Are they manipulative? Are they mean / arrogant / patronizing / a bully? Do they have basic social skills down? Are they controlling / passive-aggressive? Are they safe?

All of these (and more) 'markers' are tracked by women ... and should be shared amongst them. Women need to look after women. If someone is inept or a bully ... other women should know that.

Tracking the rep of women in the OM community is much simpler. Do they show up on time for their OMs? Are they in their right range? Do they have a good relationship with their pussy and body? Do they support other women? (See entry above "Getting References.")

Gatekeeper: in an OM community or network, a gatekeeper is someone who makes sure that persons who would likely be dangerous and / or untowardly disruptive ... do not enter the 'energetic' space of the established group. OM is about creating a safe space for a woman's sexuality to open. Women are nude from the waist down ... and in an incredibly vulnerable position ... during an OM. Sexual predators, emotionally unstable or violent individuals, and people with poor boundary skills or social skills ... have no place in an OM community ... without extensive professional support / guidance / safeguards.

The gatekeeper has historically been an "unofficial" position ... and in some communities ... the responsibility is often distributed among several individuals *who have the same ethical sensibilities.*

The only feedback necessary – to refused prospective members – is often ... "you are not a fit for our community at this time." (Getting into specifics about *why* someone is being rejected ... may lead to legal issues. And ... frequently – for untrained people – simply saying "something about [x] feels off" ... covers what is actually 'known.' Given the sensitivity of the practice and the vulnerability of the women ... a high bar of entry should be expected. No one – certainly no man – has the *right* ... to stroke a woman's pussy. She gets the final say on what happens to her body.)

Getting References [for a potential new partner / coach / trainer / class / circle]: OM is a very intimate, very vulnerable, very edgy sexual practice.

And OM is fundamentally a community-based practice. Talking and connecting with other OMers – even online – allows you tap a rich vein of experience. Consider it crowd-sourcing orgasm. Generally speaking, whatever you are encountering, grappling with, or experiencing ... there are 2 dozen other people somewhere in the world – at a minimum – who have had a similar experience ... and can offer some support / guidance.

One of the ways to lean on the OM community ... whether online and global, or in person and local ... is asking for – and giving – references. Who is a great teacher or trainer? What coaches have people *actually* used – and still strongly recommend? What new courses (and 90% of OM-elated courses should be considered "new" and "lightly" [or never] field-tested – unless they have been held, unchanged, for a minimum of 18 months) are actually half-way decent and worth the investment? Who are the outstanding strokers? Who are the experienced women OMers? Who is good with – and might be willing to train – newbies? Who prefers to OM with experienced OMers only? Who hosts great OM circles?

Be prepared to provide some information – when you are ready. How did you learn to OM: a partner showed you, you took a class (when? who led it? was it good?), you got private OM coaching (when? who with? were they any good?)? When was your first OM? How many OMs have you completed (roughly)?

A Guide to Somatic OMing

Have you OMed with more than one partner? Have you OMed at an OM circle? Is your OM practice active or dormant? How many OMs have you completed in the last month? Have you had any advanced OM training (when? who with? what kind?)? Do you have any special needs or requests?

What you will ask / be asked may include …

… *OM courses* ::

- what does the course cover … in terms of OM specifically?

- how much is the course?

- what kind of sales pressure / upselling is there?

- how long is the course?

- is there an advanced version of the course … if so, how does it connect to this course?

- what is the skill level / background of the instructor(s)?

- how is the authenticity and integrity of the instructors and organization?

- how would you rate the professionalism of the organization and instructors and staff?

- what kind of participant follow-up do they do after the course? … sales / self-care / 'other'?

- would you take another course from them? … if so, which ones and why? … if not, which ones and why?

A Guide to Somatic OMing

... *OM coaches* ::

- ✦ when did they complete their OM coach training (use these exact words)?

- ✦ what OM coaching program(s) did they take?

- ✦ who led the OM coaching program?

- ✦ were they certified as an OM coach?

- ✦ is their certification current? if yes, where can you confirm that?

- ✦ when did they have their first OM?

- ✦ how many (roughly) OMs have they completed?

- ✦ how many people total have they coached? ... this year?

- ✦ how many coaching sessions total have they done? ... this year?

- ✦ do they do live OM coaching?

A Guide to Somatic OMing

... OM circles ::

- ✦ where (general neighborhood) is it held?

- ✦ how often does it meet?

- ✦ what is the space like?

- ✦ what do the women think of the space?

- ✦ how many attendees typically show up?

- ✦ is it semi-open / closed / open ... to new participants?

- ✦ what is the OM experience range of the typical attendees?

- ✦ how are new prospects vetted / screened?

- ✦ is there a woman or man who is 'holding' the group?

- ✦ are there social activities – like potluck, etc. – the night of, or at different times?
- ✦ how does the group describe themselves, their energy, and their focus?

A Guide to Somatic OMing

... strokers ::

- ◆ do women trust them?
- ◆ are they creepy?
- ◆ are they a misogynist?
- ◆ are they a stalker-type / predator-type?
- ◆ do they show up on time ... and prepared?
- ◆ are they courteous and respectful?
- ◆ do they smell funny?
- ◆ do they show-up clean and well-groomed (nails clipped short, etc.)?
- ◆ would you trust your kids with them?
- ◆ are they stable?
- ◆ do they show up for OMs sober and not-high?
- ◆ when did they complete their OM training?
- ◆ what OM training have they had?
- ◆ who led their training?
- ◆ when did they have their first OM?
- ◆ how many (roughly) OMs total have they completed? ... this year?
- ◆ how many people have they OMed with? ... this year?
- ◆ what is the focus currently of their practice?

A Guide to Somatic OMing

◆ who recommends them? ... why?

◆ who *doesn't* recommend them? ... why?

◆ do they have any special needs or requirements or preferences?

◆ have they OMed with women on their periods?

◆ and [after OMing with them] ... would you OM with them again?

◆ what is their current right range – what can they handle?

... *women [strokees]* ::

- ◆ do they show up on time for OMs?
- ◆ would you trust your kids with them?
- ◆ are they stable?
- ◆ do they show up for OMs sober and not-high?
- ◆ when did they complete their OM training?
- ◆ what OM training have they had?
- ◆ who led their training?
- ◆ when did they have their first OM?
- ◆ how many (roughly) OMs have they completed? ... this year?
- ◆ how many people have they OMed with? ... this year?
- ◆ what is the focus currently of their practice?
- ◆ who recommends them? ... why?
- ◆ who *doesn't* recommend them? ... why?
- ◆ do they have any special needs or requirements or [container] preferences?
- ◆ and [after OMing with them] ... would you OM with them again?

The screening criteria are (of necessity) longer for strokers than for strokees. Women get to be messy ... and however they show up for an OM is fine. They needn't "dress up," put makeup on, or fuss in any way. In fact, they are encouraged to show up "messy" ... and be accepted for who they are – unlike the experience they may have in the outside world. It is part of the "sacred messy." This includes when they are on their period. A gentle heads up to their stroker is prudent ... so additional towels may be prepped.

Building a Stable of Partners: ... this is usually hows up as "building a stable of strokers." This is the idea that people – especially women – need to develop a pool of trusted knowledgable partners who they can call on to OM with. Women should have a deep pool (married or monogamous couples who do not OM outside the partnership are, naturally an exception) of trusted strokers that they can call on ... at any hour ... for as many OMs as they would like (spread out over their 'stable' of partners). This is essential in getting truly "filled up." Women have had to dial their desire back for men long enough. OM is designed to give women as much unencumbered limbic connection as their bodies require – no strings attached. And different strokers (and different women) will often elicit vastly different OMs and OM experiences. A woman's sex is a vast an uncharted terrain, easily dwarfing that of most men.

OM Crush: this is when ... a new-ish OMer (or even experienced OMers) become *flooded* with hormones after a particularly juicy OM ... and suddenly – given the intensity of intimacy shared within a mind-blowing OM – they start 'crushing' on their OM partner (like a crush in high school) ... and wondering if they "are the one." 97+% of the time – they're not. You are just high as a kite ... and it *feels* great! It's the OM. Experienced OMers (who wiped out pursuing those elusive connections in the past) know better. They know their bodies are amazing ... that that was an incredible ride. And not to screw up a great OM partnership.

Also, never make any life-changing commitments in the nest. Wait for the orgasm to cool off ... and see what the world looks like. Remember ... orgasm is just energy ... and it is *constantly* in flux.

Flagged OMer: this means an OMer – usually a man – has not "played well" with others. They have "poached" on a container, hit on partners, pressured their partner to pursue container-break activities … or just been an asshole / narcissist / creep. They are someone … people do not want to be in a nest with. A flag means … 'proceed with caution.'

OM is not a therapy … or reform school. And OM is not for everyone.

Blacklisted OMer: an OMer (90% of the time a male) who has demonstrated an unwillingness or inability to keep a solid OM container … and / or provide a safe space for other OMers. Someone who does not play well with others and / or is energetically taxing.

COMMUNITY

Global OM Community: OMers exist all across the globe. They constitute the [unofficial] Global OM Community. It is prudent for OMers to foster and control their own communities … with independent voices, channels, teachers, leaders, coaches, and discussions.

OM Community: this a more nebulous term. An OM Community is really any group of OMers who consider themselves a community … as well as any OMers in relative proximity to one another – whether physical, categorical, or online.

So … there is a global OM Community. There is the [dispersed] Warehouse Alumni Community. There is an LA OM community. There's one in NYC, one in London, one in Austin, and one in the San Francisco area. One can say there is a Parents-Who-OM Community, etc. Every established and recurring OM Circle can be considered a small OM community. The old online Chatboard was a mostly OMer Community back in 2007. And the current largest body of [mostly/partly] online OMers is a Facebook Closed Group … that, as of this writing, nearly 3000 member.

Historically, the first OM community was [probably] the [3] Brisbane Houses run by Nicole Daedone, south of San Francisco, in the tiny town of Brisbane, California. It was run by women and served women's orgasm. That grew into the iteration 5 years later … of the San Francisco Urban Retreat Center and

A Guide to Somatic OMing

Warehouse Living Space on Folsom Street. The Warehouse was an extraordinary experiment in creating a sensual community run by women, focused on researching women's orgasm.

OM remains a practice designed to source and empower women around their sex and their voice (with men serving as their supportive, flexible allies). If an OM Community exists … if it is in balance with OM … it will be led by women.

OM Circle: this is a name for a common form of group OMs. In OM Circles, a group of OMers come together in a space / room … for the purposes of doing one, two (most common), or more rounds of simultaneous OMs. OMers usually 'book' OM partners ahead of time (in some OM Circles having a partner 'booked' before the OM Circle is optional, in others it is mandatory – no partner booked, no admittance, no OM). Nests are laid out by the OMers (usually the strokers) … and everyone starts OM #1 at the same time (usually one person … typically an experienced stroker … acts as timekeeper and monitors a clock and calls out the 'begin,' '2-minute warning,' and 'time' time cues). There is a short break between OM Rounds … with some partners shifting nests to their next 'booked' OM partner.

And the cycle repeats. (OM Circles tend to start promptly on time … latecomers may not be admitted. The focus will be on creating a safe space for the women … who showed up on time.)

Some local groups may have a light social event afterwards. Potluck dinners are very popular in some areas.

OM Circles are [currently] self-organized by interested groups of OMers who live in relatively close proximity. (There some Best Practices and Worst Practices for creating a new OM Circle from scratch that I will cover that in a future work.)

'Joining' a local OM Circle usually means finding a contact for the group … who can screen and vet you … sufficiently so as to maintain the group's – and most especially the women's – safety and peace of mind. If you are a stroker and attend a local OM Circle ... be prompt, be kind, be well-mannered, be courteous, be low maintenance. If you are a woman ... be on time and ask questions; bring your pussy and your curiosity. Being an OMer and wanting to join a circle aren't always enough. The Circle has to 'want' new members, it has to like you, and has to feel that adding you is safe for the group ... and within its right range. No stranger [to the OM Circle] ... is 'entitled' to join.

Play nice. Keep a solid container. Cultivate – and deserve – a good rep (reputation). In a community of OMers, that is gold.

OM Outpost: this is an old euphemism for when a newly trained OMer is in an area all by themselves – or with only a handful of other OMers. There is no local franchise / affiliate / institution ... servicing the area ... providing OM training and support. It is ... an OM 'frontier.'

OM Houses: there have actually 4 waves of 'OM Houses.

'The first wave predated the Warehouse Phase (2006 – 2008). Going back to the turn of the century, Nicole Daedone and her students / followers lived in 3 'OM' houses in Brisbane California, a tiny community on San Francisco's outskirts. (They began as a part of the Morehouse community.) In them, Nicole and her companions OMed for extended periods and refined the parameters of the OM Model itself. These were sold in spring of 2006, after the decision to commit more fully to the San Francisco OneTaste Urban Retreat Center was made. The Warehouse space was leased / purchased some months later.

A Guide to Somatic OMing

The second wave can be considered the Warehouse Phase (2006 – 2008). While the Warehouse was being retrofitted by the volunteer efforts of the residents, a temporary set-up was created next door ... with the quick (and able) construction of queen-sized bunk beds. After several months of work the Warehouse space itself was ready. Eventually it sprawled to include a smaller space at the front of the Warehouse, the main Warehouse space, and a small extension into what was called 'Moss Street.' In addition, we maintained a separate residence a few doors down ... essentially a "normal" second story apartment.

The third wave was following the closing of the Warehouse (2008/2009). Basically, people wanted to live with other OMers and be able to OM frequently without hassles or the judgements of others. So a small hotel next door to the old Center was obtained and adapted for a few years.

The fourth wave of OM Houses slowly began to emerge after the closing of the hotel. People still wanted to live and OM communally. So ... here and there ... OM-friendly 'houses' emerged. Each of them is unique ... and self-regulating.

Warehouse: the peak of OM research occurred from June 2006 to July 2008 in downtown San Francisco. Nicole Daedone established the San Francisco Urban Retreat Center near Folsom and 7th Street early in the 2000s. The Center produced Intro to OM courses and about 3 or 4 courses that deepened the OM practitioners' OMing skill set.

In June of 2006, a couple of buildings east of the Center on Folsom, Nicole's company quietly 'opened' a semi-legal communal residence that was, in fact, a converted warehouse. This Warehouse went on to have a gender-balanced residency of 44-ish people – 22 female, 22 male. All residents were volunteers in an experiment in communal sensual living. We were all OMers ... and by living in the Warehouse ... we agreed to research OMing, sex, and intimacy. The population stayed at full occupancy ... while the actual residents fluctuated. About 12 of us were there for the whole 2 years.

After announcing the closing the Warehouse in 2008, Nicole simplified the OM teachings ... in preparation for mainstreaming OM. A lot of what we learned in the Warehouse Phase was shelved ... only for bits and pieces to be rolled out over the years to jazz up course offerings from time to time. Those 2 years still – in my opinion, as well as in the opinion of others – represent the high water mark [so far] in OM research and development.

[OM] Lineage: a lineage is a way of tracking "versions" and branches of related schools of study – whether in philosophy, martial arts, or some other modality. OM was not created in a vacuum – it was not "the immaculate invention." While the OM Model is distinct, brilliant, and in many ways revolutionary ... the primary visionary behind OM, Nicole Daedone, worked and studied in several local communities and sexual models ... that are similar structurally to OM ... before she created the OM Model. She was a part of the Morehouse community – which practices 'Doing' – for a while, and considered its leader, Vic Baranco, a personal mentor. She also spent time with the people of the (much smaller) Welcomed Consensus Community – which practices another version of clit stroking. In addition, she received advice from another master stroker, Ray Vetterlein.

* * *

A Guide to Somatic OMing

:: OM Principles ::

Right Range: this is a key concept in OM ... and has applications outside of the nest, in day-to-day living.

One of the best illustrations of 'right range' is in physical stretching. If a person doesn't sufficiently stretch, say, their hamstrings ... their running may be impaired. If they stretch too far ... they risk over-stretching and hurting themselves. The goal of the runner ... is work within their body's 'right range' for that day. Too little ... no improvement. Too much ... and likely injury. Just enough ... and they are in their 'right range' ... for that particular day. Their body is strengthened and develops / grows.

In OM, practitioners are encouraged to tune in to their bodies ... and discern what their 'right range' is for a given activity or context. And it may change over time ... and from day-to-day ... and from OM-to-OM. (Just like an individual's physical flexibility.)

So the question is asked, "What is in my right range here ... today?" Is it ...

- ✦ ... OMing in a group or privately.

- ✦ ... OMing with a familiar partner or a new person or a stranger.

- ✦ ... OMing with female or male stroker.

- ✦ ... OMing with an experienced OMer or with a brand new OMer.

- ✦ ... asking for what I want from my stroker, or bringing my approval to whatever stroke they bring.

- ✦ ... doing one OM today, or two, or three, or four, or more ...

- ✦ ... receiving OM coaching / suggestions from a woman – or a man.

- ✦ ... sharing my OM experiences with a close friend, with family, with acquaintances, with strangers ... of a specific gender.

- ✦ ... asking for help / support.

- ✦ ... asking for an OM.

- ✦ ... being asked for an OM.

- ✦ ... saying a clear 'Yes.'

- ✦ ... saying a clear 'No.'

- ✦ ... showing my pussy to a friend or to an acquaintance or to a stranger.

Part of the practice of OM is to learn to ask for (within the constraints of the OM container) what one wants. Distinguishing right range is key to doing that responsibly. We know more about ourselves ... than a stranger is likely to.

Riding the Wave: in OM this usually refers to "riding the wave" ... of a woman's orgasm – and is something that both strokee and stroker do. It is a central tenet of OM.

Havingness Level: When I learned to OM (2006), 'Havingness Level' was a core concept to the practice.

In it's simplest terms, our personal mythos – the story we tell ourselves about who we are (and who we *can* be) in the world – determines how much 'good stuff' – pleasure, connection, approval, intimacy, love, orgasm, 'fun,' etc. – we think we deserve / are allowed.

Now the curious part is ... when we reach that magic level ... we will arrange to turn that spigot off. We will drive away our partners, start fights, isolate ourselves, become thoroughly unpleasant to be around (or some other "fix") – all to avoid "having too much" (or "more than our 'quota'").

The practice of OM is partially about bumping up against our invisible ceilings ... and, through staying present in our OMs ... *raising* that particular ceiling. We literally rewrite our personal mythos.

Women, in particular, have been conditioned – mercilessly – by our culture ... to "dial themselves down," to not be "too much." "Don't be too turned on, too expressive, too big with their energy, too dominant, too demanding for sex / orgasm / pleasure."

OM gradually loosens the top of that kettle ... and reintroduces the OMer to their own body, and to a more authentic range of _____ [insert whatever they have been rationing for themselves].

Havingness Level — *Some Rough Seas* ::

When a new OMer encounters their havingness level in a particular area (say ... orgasm) ... their first reaction is often discomfort ... "oh, that's not me ... [putting their hands up] sorry." Discomfort, awkwardness, alarm ... can all signify an old crusty ceiling ... is – surprise! – flexible after all.

Rather than being a cause for rejoicing (for some) ... it is often experienced as a cause for alarm. Your very identity is ... shifting / changing / unstable / threatened / questioned. Malleable.

And ... that's ... okay.

OT historically has encouraged people to plunge right ahead.

You get to choose.... whether to continue ... and how fast to go. If you wipe out, OT will throw up their hands and say ... "we're just an entertainment company" ... and you will have to pick yourself up ... and clean up any messes you made.

So ... check in with *your* body ... get support from other OMers (ask questions) ... and set the pace *you* want. And expect bumps ...

... and some growing pains.

Havingness Level — *Going Meta* ::

Once you get the concept of 'havingness levels' and start noticing where they show up around OMs (asking for OMs – making requests – is a big one for many people), ... you will start spotting them in non-OMing areas: relationships, family, job, hobbies, finances.

And that's a big deal. Pat yourself on the back (give yourself approval for growing & learning).

OMing will help you recognize how your body reacts around – or 'implements' – a havingness level.

It's okay to recognize that your entire family has a level of [x] in the area of fun / finances / authenticity / connection.

Havingness levels are just unconscious scripts ... that we have been inadvertently renewing each day. Becoming conscious of a level ... introduces choice. And ... the prospect of play.

You ... and the world ... aren't as stingy as you thought.

You can have more.

Put Attention On [Person X]: this was shorthand for ... being *fully present* and energetically engaged with another person. "Put attention of Chris." This was a skill we cultivated [in the Warehouse years]. It is a natural extension of OM – where the stroker ... puts their [full] attention ... on the strokee.

It is not merely feigning interest – the "being fully present" part takes care of that.

A Guide to Somatic OMing

Bringing Approval (as opposed to 'conditional approval'): in OM a stroker "brings" their approval ... to whatever the strokee generates. In other words ... (using the masculine pronoun) he doesn't 'wait' to see what shows up ... and how he feels about it. He generates and 'brings' his unconditional approval ... to the OM ... and to her pussy. She farts ... he approves. She weeps ... he approves. She rages ... he approves. She has pussy farts ... he approves. She has a very heavy menstrual flow ... he approves. She is dead silent ... he approves. In this sense, 'approval' is a somatic address ... a somatic field. And she gets to spend the OM *in* it.

Sometimes, that is the most impactful contribution a stroker will bring to an OM – simply being unconditionally 'approving' of a woman ... for ... 15 ... minutes.

Bring Your Approval: this is very much a specific state or attitude. It is possible ... when a person I am with does [x] ... to silently a) disapprove, b) be completely neutral, or c) bring my approval. When I am stroking a woman ... if she cries out, I bring my approval (silently). If she farts, I bring my approval (silently). If she starts swearing, I bring my approval (silently).

Bring Your Full Attention: this is pretty much what it says. No planning your car route home. No wondering how the local basketball team is doing at the moment. Bring your full attention ... and keep it on her pussy and her orgasm ... for 15 minutes. This is the 'meditation' part. Show up. Fully.

Be Present: ... is the state of not being distracted or inside talking with oneself. It means being fully in one's body ... centered and with your attention focused outward ... on your partner. Women – especially in an OM – can detect when their partner "checks out" or has "wandering attention-itus." Your attention (as a stroker) impacts the OM.

Being Acknowledged: one of the many highly valued somatic addresses or states in OM ... is "being acknowledged." Some of us take it for granted ... but settling down for an OM – and ignoring your partner – is a big faux pas. It is an integral part of connecting with another human being. You can acknowledge your partner by [briefly] making eye contact – and being present – before an OM starts. ... or by actually "hearing" their requests ... and signaling that you heard them – by saying "thank you." Being acknowledged is a fundamentally different somatic experience (feeling in your body) ... than being ignored. The best strokers are masters at acknowledgement ... and the timing / duration / intensity / communication channel etc. of those acknowledgements.

Getting Filled Up: At its most basic level, an OM is designed to support women in "filling up" ... with a much needed type of energetic nourishment: sensual limbic connection with another human being ... with that person's full attention, and with unconditional approval. The state of culture in the west is such that ... most women are not touched *with approval* enough, their sex is often rudely dismissed as secondary in importance to men's orgasm and pleasure, and their partners rarely give the woman's sex their full undivided attention. As a result, most women are "parched" somatically ... and get by with their "connection" well or tank ... dangerously low or empty. The practice of OM allows women to "get filled up" and become "hydrated."

It can take 2 years or more for a woman with an 'active' OM practice (12+ OMs per week) ... to get "filled up." And that state ... being "filled up" is a very definite state or somatic address. Women who reach it ... report noticing that their body has shifted ... that their bodies are no longer running checks in the background ... wondering where the next 'fix' of limbic intimacy is going to come from. They can feel their bodies relax ... and open up. Their field of awareness becomes much larger ... and they often experience a [new] feeling of curiosity about their world.

Men who stroke women ... are nourished as well ... through being in the field of a woman's orgasm regularly. They may experience a different kind of "filling up." The disparity of what men can get and what women are 'allowed' in the west ... is huge, however. There are other practices that can address men's other energetic or limbic needs. OM is designed to address and correct a cultural imbalance (and deficit) most women experience – and have had to put up with.

A Guide to Somatic OMing

OM is designed – and reserved specifically – for … helping end the cultural drought … for limbic connection in women's lives. A woman has the inalienable right to ask for an OM … be stroked … and then get up and go about her day … owing her partner *nothing.*

Sacred Messy: OM means embracing the 'sacred messy.' (This was the only time the practice mentioned anything *remotely* related to religion, god, or spirituality.) In the context of OM, the Sacred Messy means … the multitude of fluids, noises, odors … that a woman's body might "release" during an OM. The founder of OM made a point of strongly emphasizing that … in the course of her OM practice … "every fluid, noise, and odor a woman's body *could* make" … she had made. And if it was okay for her to do [x] … then, by golly, it was okay for any other woman who OMs to do it. Not just 'okay,' but fabulous … these were all manifestations of a woman's 'messy' orgasm. It was her birthright.

And as strokers, we were trained that things could get messy, to roll with it, *and* to bring our unconditional approval to our partner. The best strokers were often not the best looking guys (or gals) … but the ones who got this idea and fully mastered it.

Following the Energy: this is a core concept in OM. [in an OM] the stroker is instructed … to "follow the energy" in the OM. When the stroker is doing upstrokes … there will come a moment … when the energy 'shifts' … and 'wants' to go down. Experienced strokers will 'feel' the shift coming … and … right before the energy actually flips … they will 'change direction' of the stroke.

Another example is after the OM … a stroker having done some grounding pressure … may 'notice' that the woman's body may need more grounding … and asks the woman … "do you want more / different grounding?" (The woman will often have specific grounding directions … just for that OM … angle / location / intensity / etc.)

OMing gradually teaches both the woman and her stroker how to read energy. That transfers outside of the nest. You can follow the energy in a conversation or a room full of people ... just as well as in an OM. There are expansions and contractions ... 'flat' periods ... 'stuck' energy ... 'blocked energy' ... and nice peaks.

Vigilance Center: this a core OM concept. To OM a woman must be able to relax and be able to receive the strokes her partner brings to her. Every task a stroker takes on ... is one less that she has to manage – *if* her 'vigilance center' trusts the stroker. Stroking a woman whose body ... is rigid with alarm / fear / concern ... is unlikely to lead to her connecting with her orgasm.

Part of the reason OM was created ... was to be able to offer women support for connecting with her own body, her own sex / pussy, and her own voice – in safety. Women today live in a society ... where (most of them) have to be constantly vigilant for risks, threats, and dangers – most of which, unfortunately, will be posed by men. The part of their mind that is never off ... that is constantly monitoring risks in the background ... in OM is called the 'vigilance center.'

The OM Container ... was created specifically to give women a safe space to chill in. That is why it is so important that the container be held and rigorously honored by her stroker. When a woman's body / pussy *knows* that her stroker is solid and trustworthy ... that they have her back – without question – than ... than they can begin to relax into an 'open state.'

She wants to go there. You just have to demonstrate – consistently – that she can count on you.

Talk to Your Pussy: this is a simple, yet profound idea for many women.

Actually talk ... to your pussy. Establish a relationship. Ask it questions. Run things by it. Build up rapport. Rebuild trust. Look after it. Care for it. Honor it.

A Guide to Somatic OMing

Your pussy is more than just a strong case of the hornys. It pays attention to *everything.* And it likely knows who is lying ... and who will have your back. In older times, a woman's pussy was a source of an ancient, deep, respected wisdom.

Talk to your pussy.

And this goes for men as well. When you are in relationship with a woman ... talk to her pussy – respectfully. Build rapport with it. And *never* betray it.

"Stroke for Your Own Pleasure:" this is a key concept within OM. It means that – **while keeping a strong container and while meeting any request your strokee makes that you can fulfill** – a stroker should tune into their own body ... and stroke the woman in a way that is pleasurable to them (the stroker).

Listen to Your Pussy: this is advice given to women who OM. More broadly, it is an invitation to foster a deeper connection with a woman's own native intuition, desires, and body sense / wisdom. Women are often asked to address their pussy directly – aloud or silently – and notice what intuitions / hunches / communications arise. A big part of the design of OM ... is restoring a woman's voice, a woman's intuition, and ... yes ... a woman's sex to a position of honor and esteem within a community.

What a woman wants sexually matters.

* * *

:: OM Concepts ::

Open Up: this is a subtle, complex term. It basically means ... to be able to relax ... and unclench what has been clenched ... unlock what has been locked (physically) ... to be able to allow energy to flow freely. It means it is safe enough that barriers can be lowered and defenses relaxed. It can apply to either stroker or strokee.

The OM Container is designed to create a solid zone of safety and security ... so that a woman's body ... can relax fully ... and eventually 'open up.' Her first 50 to 120 OMs will often just be her body getting relaxed about the OM Container, OM, and her partner(s).

As a general rule, you don't tell a woman "to open up."* You create a safe space for her sex and her body and treat her with elevated levels of respect. Eventually ... when her body is satisfied it is not a trick or a hoax ... she begins to 'open up' energetically. All of this impacts her ability to connect with and enjoy her orgasm. It is also *deeply* linked to her willingness to authentically express herself in the world.

(*The sole possible exception to "telling a woman to open up" ... is when she has *expressly* requested coaching from an *experienced* OM Coach (not a 'hack') ... and usually a woman coach. Men as a cardinal rule ... should avoid *ever* telling a woman what to do with her orgasm. Ever.)

Metabolizing [an OM]: this is a rich limbic term. Just as a cortex (logical) mind may organize and tidy up a room filled with new objects ... so too will a limbic system "process" somatically (in the body) ... any new experiences (including emotions, sensations, or energies) it had in an OM. The word 'metabolize' is used because the process is akin to digestion ... with energy being freed in the body as different experiences are assimilated into the body's stored maps.

A Guide to Somatic OMing

In some instances, physical labor or activity – doing the dishes, cleaning a floor, or working in the garden – aids this "processing." Most of these tasks leave the cortex [mind] in neutral ... and require the person to be 'in' their body ... during the activity – hence, they are perfect for aiding somatic processing.

No "Get-Off:" this can refer to when a strokee is refusing every stroke the stroker has at their disposal. There is no perceptible turn-on to work with. It is there ... but it is being withheld. It is just one of many somatic addresses that can arise in an OM. (See the term "Taking the Finger Off" below.)

New strokers with less than 500 OMs ... should not even attempt to distinguish this. There is a substantial risk of getting caught in head games with themselves. Just stroke ... take the strokee's adjustments gracefully ... pay attention ... bring your unconditional approval.

"Taking the Finger Off:" this is again one of those terms which has a specific meaning inside an OM ... and a metaphoric one outside of OM.

In OMs, sometimes a stroker ... gets 'lost' energetically. An option of *last* resort ... is to remove the finger from the clit (after safeporting their partner). This happened rarely (during the Warehouse days) ... and mostly when a stroker was inundated with 'adjustments' from their strokee ... faster than they could follow. It allows a reset to occur ... and the energy to settle a bit. The stroker would hold themselves still ... concentrate on even breaths ... and ... when they were ready and felt a connection again ... resume stroking.

Occasionally (and even more rarely) the stroker is "lost" ... because the strokee is refusing every stroke you have at your disposal ... in which case, pausing or taking your finger off *is* an option. This is called ... 'taking your finger off if there's no get-off.'

(Note: this is *not* meant as a 'tool' to control the woman. Rather ... it was a practical measure when the stroker got hopelessly lost. Remember ... the woman feels *everything* – so continuing the OM with a stroker that is "lost" can be excruciating for the women as well.**)**

Outside of OMs, "taking the finger off" was a metaphor ... for when an interaction (e.g., a conversation or relationship) had become too expensive energetically. We would "take our finger off" by stopping speaking or interacting with the other party. If they were a member of the OM community ... we would simply say "I'm taking my finger off now." This was a way to signal our [conversation] partner ... in a value-neutral way ... that the interaction was taking more of our energy / bandwidth than we wanted to spend at that moment, on that topic. Basically ... what they were doing to connect with us ... wasn't working.

The smart ones adapted ... and changed *how* they communicated. Next time.

Resistance*: this is a complex term. In OM culture, resistance can be most easily understood as an argument ... an argument between someone and their body, or between parts of their body, or between someone and their coach / teacher, or between their body (pussy) and the coach / teacher.

Resistance isn't necessarily bad. It is friction, tension ... energy locked up at the moment. At its most basic ... it is the body's way of protecting itself ... often (though not always) in the face of information coming in *very* fast ... or that seems to be contradictory.

In a woman (strokee), resistance most often shows up as ... fighting with her pussy or turn-on. The body does what it does and responds naturally. She may have ideas (either personal or culturally-based, or both) about what 'responses' are "good" (approved) or "bad" (scandalous, shameful, etc.). She may lie down for an OM ... and decide that she is feeling *too* much pleasure – or responding *too* enthusiastically – or not "enough." If she is wary of feeling (or showing) "too much" ... she will often 'dial down' her desires / turn-on. Her stroker will be dutifully working to increase the energy ... while she is applying the brakes. This is one example of resistance.

In a stroker (often male), resistance most often shows up as ... reluctance to follow the requests of the stroker ... or unwillingness to follow the energy (the energy wants to go down – a lot – but he wants the energy to go up ... and tries to "make" it go up). This is another example of resistance. Strokers ... in OM, her pussy / orgasm leads. Always. Get with the program.

(*A note of caution: this term has been misapplied and misused by some OM instructors and coaches. Sometimes you are resisting the coaching – and sometimes it is just bad coaching – and resistance is a wise response on the part of the body. Use – and receive – any 'coaching' with caution.)

"Processing:" when the air quotes' version was used ... this form of "processing" referred to a much disparaged tendency to "talk about experiences in order to reach a satisfying intellectual understanding of an experience." In 2006, most Warehouse residents, when they moved in, were habituated "processors." A "processor" would take an experience that lasted 15 minutes ... and then spend 4 hours analyzing it in conversations with others ... about that experience 'meant.' They would also 'pull' others into "processing" with them. "What do you think that meant??" Their conversation would often include large amounts of ... "then I said ... then he said ... then she said ...." This kind of "processing" was very much intellectually based ... and men were very susceptible to it.

Gradually, under Nicole's patient tutelage ... we learned to "get out of our heads" (the male model of the world) and "back into our bodies" (the female model of the world). OM was a key part of this. Why talk about one OM for 4 hours ... when you could have another 6+ OMs? Gradually, each person came to see the intellectualizations ... were just extended periods of becoming disconnected from our bodies ... and that they almost *never* produced anything actionable. Mostly, they were a way of "peacocking" intellectually – ironically enough, for the attentions of the women. Instead of stroking them, we talked about what stroking 'meant' – and how we [men] would "organize" it more efficiently.

Instead of endlessly replaying small bits of our lives on a intellectual "VCR" ... we learned (gradually) to *stay in* the experience, connect with our partners, and to really *feel* them. It got so that ... when a new person started processing

… we would just say, "you're processing…" and walk away. We learned to tell … when someone was *in* their body and speaking a core personal truth / experience. *That* we listened to.

It was a start.

Trigger(s): in the context of OM, 'triggers' refer to 'trauma triggers.' This was an acknowledgement that OMs could.occasionally stir shit up. When an old trauma gets 'triggered,' the body often goes into a state of high alert and adrenalized alarm … exactly as if a danger was immediately present.

Trauma: OM has a problematic relationship to trauma. While it is true that OM has aided many people in resolving and metabolizing past traumas, it has also been over-recommended to people … who needed more trained support around their existing past traumas. As a result, it has messed some people up. There was a cavalier attitude during the Warehouse years to trauma. The strong got stronger … and the weak were discarded. And once the support of community was ended with the closing of the Warehouse … that tendency merely intensified.

As a result, OM exists today [in many communities] largely without any significant foundation or protocols … for recognizing and supporting appropriately … people at risk from either old traumas being retriggered … or new traumas occurring. This is a *huge* gap in the OM community and the OM culture overall and needs to be fully addressed in the coming years.

Lastly, through a mixture of rough / poor handling and support … new traumas have occurred as a result of OM trainings and coaching. A disturbing proportion of OM trainers … are pretty messed up … and many have gone into therapy as a result.

OM continues to be an amazing resource for many people. But the deficit in training and support around recognizing and responding appropriately to trauma and trauma cues … is currently enormous.

A Guide to Somatic OMing

Assigned Author(ship): this is term means making someone else the "assigned author" of something you (or someone else) actually did. You did 'x' ... but you give the credit (or the blame) to someone else. It is a way of mis-coding / deflecting / avoiding agency. When people first come to OM, both women *and* men often have a script in their heads ... that says, "a woman's orgasm is the man's responsibility." It is not. It is the woman's responsibility – and part of her expression. The most a man can do ... is partner with her ... and assist her in whatever way she requests him to. She is the sole agent / author of her orgasm.

Statement of Desire: part of the OM practice is connecting with our bodies and learning to speak our desires ... cleanly, clearly, and powerfully. Expression is part of our power, our agency. It is vital – and an integral part of OM – to understand that *speaking* a [statement of] desire ... is *not* the same as ... making a request to have that desire fulfilled.

Desires are separate and distinct from requests, although many people mistakenly collapse them. (See the Note 'Desire & Request' for more background.)

Intention: this is one of the more complex OM concepts. In OM ... we say "set an intention." This is a very similar to mentally "rehearsing" skiing or another physical sport. Studies have shown that "imagining" an activity ... lights up many of the same areas of the brain ... as doing the actual activity does. Similarly, if you mentally "intend" upstrokes ... and change *nothing* in how you are *actually* stroking ... your partner (the strokee) will often experience your strokes as 'upstrokes' – regardless of the actual physical direction of the strokes. This is a bit trippy. You just 'think' your intention ... the body (usually) sorts it out at an energetic level.

Some of the common intentions that may be 'set' in an OM are ...
'up' (upstrokes) or 'down' (downstrokes), and 'grounding' (in the last few minutes of an OM).

Setting an Intention: in OM practitioners often "set intentions." These aren't goals per se. More like committing to a "sustained focus of awareness." If you had lost someone recently … you might set an intention for a given OM … to 'explore grief.'

'Setting an Intention' is a way of dialoguing with your body … and saying, "I'd really like to check out [x] in this OM" … and then 'letting go.' The body (or pussy) will bring up or shift your energy – or not. It is a way OM helps people explore their numinous connection … to Jung's unconscious.

"No-Commerce" Model: in the west, partnered sex (as opposed to solo sex, aka, masturbation) is frequently commerce-based. This means people run the following kind of calculation in their heads … when navigating sexual acts … "if I do [x] for her … then she has to do [z] for me." Additionally – in the US in particular – both [heteronormative] men and women often have a strong cultural bias that puts pleasing a man as more important than pleasing a woman.

OM is a 'no-commerce' model. This means this is a sex act … that is asymmetric. A woman is stroked by a partner. Period. There is no … "in-order-to-get-x." The stroker has the experience of stroking a woman in orgasm. Nothing else. There is no … "but she will make-out / have sex / 'put out' later for me." Or you are doing it wrong.

OM has been carefully designed to create a safe space to support empowering women around *their* sex and *their* voice.

There are other activities / sex acts where a man can be the focus of both partners.

'Demo' (Demonstration of a Woman in Orgasm): these were relatively common once, then stopped, and now appear to have returned.

A 'demo' is a public display of 'stroking a woman to orgasm.' It is – literally – a demonstration. It is *not,* however, a public demonstration of OM. Techniques

A Guide to Somatic OMing

and strokes that would be container violations in OM ... may be used freely in a demo. And generally ... the demo is not fixed in length. It might be scheduled / promoted to be a half an hour or an hour in length ... and end up being some other length, depending on how it unfolds. (The woman may have more / less energy (orgasm) than anticipated.)

Demos are intended to give non-OMers a taste of what the landscape of a woman's orgasm may look like ... and give them a taste of what it feels like to be in a limbic field. (And it is also a sales tool for institutions.) The audience for the demo may vary in size – it might be as few as 6 or as many as 40. In addition to the woman (usually on an elevated massage table) and her stroker, there is usually one person – an experienced OMer – narrating and explaining what transpires. Frames are explained and audience members are encouraged to call out sensations in their body as they feel them. In the past, at a certain point in the demo ... audience members have been encouraged to come up (one at a time) and stand next to the woman being stroked ... and even, on occasion, to touch their shin ... and "get a feel of the energy flowing through her body." Also, the audience is sometimes encouraged to ask questions directly ... of the woman being stroked. The emcee frequently ... clarifies and repeats back ... the sometimes whispered / muffled answers.

There was actual Demo Training in the past – for both strokees and strokers. It actually takes a bit of skill, experience, and turn-on to ... project the energy out ... enough that it is palpable to the audience. Often, during the Warehouse days ... the most turned-on woman in the community was chosen to do that week's demo. They were schooled in how to build and hold energy / turn-on ... prior to the demo. It was not uncommon for the demo woman ... to get up on the massage table ... already in visible abdominal contractions. It is a skill ... and they were very good. Their strokers were trained to get everything out of the way energetically ... and fully support the woman's turn-on ... 'flowering.'

In the past, the Warehouse leadership had strict warnings for any graduates ... who gave "unauthorized" demos. Really ... this was for 3 reasons: one, a 'screwed up' demo would reflect badly on OM – and attract unwanted attention

A Guide to Somatic OMing

(from the press and presumably – depending on how big the 'screw-up' was – law enforcement); two, it actually takes a lot of planning, expertise, forethought, and (most importantly) screening and security to do it right; and three, avoiding any brand dilution for institutions offering OM training.

In the last few years, OMers have begun to get comfortable doing 'informal demos' ... really, of OM ... to small handfuls of people they know well. And this is healthy. OM should be shared responsibly ... and where possible ... free of commercial caveats.

Pussy Orientation: In the early stages of a woman's OM training during the Warehouse Days ... she was encouraged to actually look at her pussy – in the presence of other women in her class. And bring her approval to her pussy. And she was encouraged ... gently ... to set aside vague and concealing euphemisms ... in favor of saying – loud and proud – 'pussy' when referring to her own ... or other women's sex. (See the entry above for "pussy.")

Another form of this occurs when some experienced women OMers ... who have had experiences with first-time strokers having difficulty finding their way around their pussy (locating a small clit, navigating a complex hood, etc.) ... take the initiative and give a new stroker a pre-OM Pussy Orientation. This allows the stroker to ask questions, get a good look at what her pussy actually looks like ... and generally ... get oriented. The tour can be "observe-only" or with "full glove" contact ... whatever the woman feels comfortable with. It can be part of the process of reclaiming her sex.

Note: at present, this is not a part of OM ... and partners should be safeported and asked whether they wish to do this. The option should only be initiated by women.

Group OMs: it is common in many [unofficial] OM communities ... for OMers to practice together. A group OM is most frequently structured as an OM Circle. In an OM Circle, OMers will gather at a specific location at a specific date and time ... typically one that has a large open common room big enough for all the OMers and their nests. Depending on the location and number of OMing pairs ... some nest materials may need to be brought to the location. Typically, if people take the time to come together to OM, they will do 2 or more rounds of OM. Nests are laid out – taking care to not have them be too close to each other. A timekeeper is chosen or volunteers (usually one of the more experienced strokers) and each round of OMs starts when everybody is ready ... and the timekeeper says, "Begin."

When the OMs are completed, people may stay and connect, share experiences, and ask for tips. Some OM Circles have a potluck dinner afterwards ... as a way of socializing.

OMing in groups can be a bit daunting for some more quiet types. Generally, OMers are not asked to "quiet down" for the sake of newbies' nerves. The practice is orgasmic meditation ... and the intention is support women connecting to their sex – and their voices. It can take some people a few OMs to settle into their bodies. Group OMs are not for everyone. Stay in your right range. Don't force it.

The primary advantage of group OMs are 2: first, you learn faster. Your body is picking up a *huge* amount of information while OMing ... from the 4 (or 5 or 6...) other pairs of people OMing at the same time. Your focus will (should) be on your partner. But your body will hear things from other nests ... sounds ... adjustments ... requests ... and go, "I didn't know that was possible ...." Second, the energy dynamic in a room of group OMs will be richer, more complex, with more dynamics. It is like listening to – and feeling – an orchestra. Again ... your body will sense things ... and make new, subtle distinctions. Plus you may have a chance to ask – or answer – questions of other practitioners / strokers / strokees.

OM is fundamentally a community-based practice. We learn from – and support – each other's OM practice.

Switching (Rotating) Nests: this may occur in group OMs (OM circles) ... when there is more than one round of OMs.

A Guide to Somatic OMing

In the Warehouse days, we had 2 rounds of morning group OMs. After the first round of OMing was complete, the strokers would get up (gracefully and quietly) and move to their next OM partner – and to that partner's [OM] nest. As a rule, rotating is done only by strokers, never by strokees (the women).

OM Kit: experienced strokers who travel to OM with their partners often do so with an OM Kit they keep handy and freshly stocked. A typical OM kit will have … 2 types of gloves in the stroker's preferred size (in case they OM with a woman allergic to one of the glove materials), a jar of <u>OneStroke</u> lube, a small supply of [fresh] coconut oil (in case their partner is sensitive to one of the OneStroke ingredients), a couple of clean washcloths (to act as OM towels) in a clean sandwich-size bag (to keep them sanitary), a small digital timer with a large number display (for easy reading), a couple of empty sandwich bags (to stash used OM towels), and a small bottle of baby powder (in case the gloves don't go on easily). These should be kept in a breathable bag (to prevent mildewing), like an <u>Eagle Creek bag</u>. Care should be taken to keep the OM Kit clean at all times and stocked with fresh supplies.

A well-stocked OM Kit means a woman just needs to provide her pussy and a mat and some cushions … and an OM can take place.

Some strokers who have cars may have cushions and a [clean] portable nest as well.

In dense populations of OMers, (like parts of San Francisco) a prepared stroker may have an opportunity to do a couple of "spontaneous" OMs a week – or even a day. ("Hi ___. Are you free for an OM in an hour? I have time for one OM before my meeting.") While most of the OM Kit contents may not be used for any given OM … carrying one signals potential strokees … that you are an attentive stroker and can be counted on to come prepared – and it signals a commitment to provide a solid experience / container for the strokee's partners.

[the] Involuntary: OMers talk about the [strokee's] body going "into the involuntary" … like it's a place. We will also say, "activating the involuntary." What this means, in practice is … that we (either the strokee or stroker) notice

A Guide to Somatic OMing

physical changes that are typically associated with involuntary physiological processes ... such as pussy contractions (external or internal), pussy lip engorgement, and abdominal spasms. Some of the physiology markers are associated with climax, others with pre-climax states. The signs noted are not [normally] subject to conscious control ... hence, the use of word, 'involuntary.'

Which is a long way of saying ... the body is now doing its own thing ... and at least part of what we observe – as either strokee or stroker – is not being generated by our cortex-mind. The limbic system is at play.

Limbic Connection: this is a complex term, one best experienced ... rather than explained. That said ... limbic connection in an OM ... occurs when the natural physiological mirroring processes kick in ... and both participants' limbic systems sync up across multiple biologic and electrical subsystems.

The unconscious mirroring of unique physical attributes / signifiers – pulse, respiration, posture, speech volume and cadence – is one of the hallmarks of biologic rapport. This can occur at deeper levels in OM. OMers share sensate frames at the conclusion of every OM ... and frequently, their internal experiences sync up ... often in uncanny ways.

One of the core assertions / assumptions in the OM Model ... is that humans need limbic connection ... not merely touch ... but a deeper resonance with another human being. OM is designed to fill at least some of that need.

Limbic System: this is a rich, central term in OM. According to Wikipedia, "... [t]he limbic system supports a variety of functions including emotion, behavior, motivation, long-term memory, and olfaction. Emotional life is largely housed in the limbic system, and it has a great deal to do with the formation of memories."

In OM, the limbic system is contrasted with its 'opposite' ... the cortex system. Roughly speaking, within the OM culture ... this is pitched as the limbic system is the unconscious, primitive, intuitive 'mind' ... and its counterpart is the more logical, reason-based cortex-mind. It's important to note ... that the use of Limbic System with OM is more of a mythic (invented) construct ... than a use of a strict scientific definition of the term.

A central theme of the OM Model is learning to operate – for extended periods of time – exclusively from the "desire-based" limbic system ... as an alternative to the rational cortex system. And to extend to it equal, if not greater, value ... in making both day-to-day decisions, as well as major life decisions. This sometimes referred to as "living a desire-based life."

Cortex [System]: in OM the cortex [system] is shorthand for the thinking part of the mind and is contrasted with the limbic [system]. In western culture, men are often rewarded for cortex-based skills ... talking, analyzing, organizing, calculating, critiquing, problemsolving, ... and more generally, 'mansplaining.'

One of the first things men new to OM try to do when they enter the OM community / culture ... is try to organize it 'better' or explain women's orgasm to women or explain how we are "doing it all wrong." It is best to think of it as an unconscious 'tic.' The men who become good strokers learn to quiet their chatter ... and open up to their limbic system. The rest eventually wander off. (See also, *'[Intellectual] Peacocking.'*)

OM is designed to foster and deepen our connections to our own limbic system ... as well as support us in connecting better with the limbic systems of others. (Limbic system can be simplified here and considered as ... our intuition and body wisdom.)

Getting [OM] Training: the gateways to beginning an OM practice vary widely. Some people read Nicole Daedone's explanation of it in her book, "Slow Sex," and use that alone to start a practice with a partner. Other people watch the OneTaste videos on YouTube ... and use that to start with. Still others have taken one of the online OM orientation classes from OneTaste (OT). Some people were shown ("trained") by a partner who was an experienced OMer. And some people received hands-on training in OT's old classes or from OT-trained-and-sometimes-certified OM coaches. It varies.

A Guide to Somatic OMing

The phrase 'get training' is generally a directive to get more complete, more formal OM training. This is often a requirement for joining private OM groups ("OM circles"). Basically, formal training makes sure everyone is on the same page ... and knows how to OM – and how to behave / be a courteous OMer. Some women want to OM only with partners who have been well / thoroughly trained – and vetted (by trainers / coaches).

The culture of OM is quite complex ... and there is a lot to learn. Much of it consists of a particular etiquette that OMers rely on when participating in such a vulnerable practice. Some of that is conveyed in the book, "Slow Sex," and some is not. (And some parts of "Slow Sex" are out of date.) Additionally, how OM was taught has varied ... year to year and class to class. There appear to be more than a dozen or so ... slightly different OM "models" ... in the wild.

The current institutional offerings of OM training are in flux. In recent years, Certified OM Coaches ... often had more class time ... than actual experience OMing ... which has led to reports of mediocre-to-awful OM coaching experiences. Caveat emptor.

Bottom line: be alert ... ask good questions ... check with the community ... use the buddy system ... be safe. Never assume a new partner has been taught the 'exact' same OM model you were. Talk to them. When in doubt ... go with what the strokee (woman) feels safest with.

OM Lab: this was a follow-up to the Introduction to OM Classes in the past. The OM Class covered the theory of OM and explained the practice of OM and addressed questions and concerns. The OM Lab (circa 2007) was a chance for students who had just completed the OM Class to actually OM ... under the supervision and guidance of experienced OMers. Live OM coaching took place – by people who actually knew OM well *and* had a lot of OMs under their belt. The OM coaches or 'guides' would walk around and offer suggestions and adjustments to the brand-new OMers. Their skill and timing would often speed up a new OMer's establishment of their OM practice tremendously. Live OM coaching remains the strongest model of OM knowledge transmission.

In particular, the guidance of senior women practitioners ... supporting and assisting new women learning how to OM was a joy to watch. I'd like to see OM Labs (possibly free / all-volunteer) come back into vogue. These would be run by experienced women OMers, supported by men, and designed to help the community foster shared learning and discovery.

OM is a community-based practice. And OM expertise and discoveries should continue to be crowd-sourced, easy to access and share safely, and transparent.

OM Journal: I recommend every beginning (and seasoned) OMer keep a private OM Journal. Record anything that stood out for you – good or bad – and especially any frames from the OM and any new discoveries – or re-discoveries. Human growth and development can be a subtle and tricky thing ... and many OMers – when they chance upon a year-old post or entry talking about an OM they had – are astonished to realize how much has shifted / opened / changed for them.

In this tech and social media age ... there are a couple of things to keep in mind.

One: your private OM 'journal' can be a mix of writings, selfies, audio recordings, and video entries. Some OMers prefer to do a quick video recording using their iPhone ... capturing the details and the energy of the [recently completed] OM. Some women have done a series of before-and-after selfies – of their face ... or of their pussy – as a way of learning more abut how their body responds to OM ... over the course of a year. These recordings / entries are very intimate and very personal – share them wisely / prudently. Avoid naming names. Use pet names or initials ... in case it ever is leaked. (I recommend only showing people an excerpt ... never the actual journal itself.)

Two: we live in a turbulent time with growing uncertainties about our privacy and sexual rights. I recommend always recording yourself alone, in private ... and always on your own device, one that is managed and controlled by you. It can get complicated (legally) if someone helpfully takes a picture of your vulva. Many details of a private OM journal entry ... can become problematic ... if it

A Guide to Somatic OMing

gets out in the world with your name on it. It's a pain, but all OMers should learn about encryption, smartphone security, malware, the cloud, and privacy / security Best Practices. They change constantly, by the way. Consider this a form of the 'digital STIs' conversation. (See Lifehacker: iPhone + Android ... for some tips.)

* * *

A Guide to Somatic OMing

:: Guidance ::

"Bring Your Attention Back…:" this is a communication for the woman to give a stroker *only.* A woman being stroked in an OM can go wherever she wants with her attention. Period. Her stroker may, however, have their attention "wander off." This can be very disruptive to an OM … and may be experienced by the woman as a [somatic] break in connection. And … since this is a practice … it can happen a lot with new strokers. There is a *lot* for them to feel / experience sometimes … and they may "check out" occasionally when the intensity gets too much. And that is okay. The woman calls them back by saying either "bring your attention back" or "where did you go?" or "where are you?" (No "please" is necessary. They have enough to do by spreading their legs.)

Nothing Extra: this is a central tenet of OM. It's a reminder that the practice should remain at its most simplest … allowing us to cut through the debris and noise of day-to-day experience: focus on the point where the finger touches the clit. OM is about reconnecting to your body … at the level of raw, un-tweaked sensation.

A list of extras new people often want to tack on to OM: music, prayers, make-up & elaborate clothes, mentions of god and goddesses (this is an unwanted and unnecessary distraction to nondeists), hugs, kisses, make-outs, flattery and fawning ("your pussy is sooo gorgeous"), horsetrading (see entry on "horsetrading"). All of these 'extras' … become yet another layer of cultural trappings to navigate through: … "do I approve or not?" and "Should I tell them what I think … or not?"

The point of the OM practice is get back to fundamentals … and connect *directly* to the body … at the level of sensation. So remember … 'nothing extra.' Come back to the stroke.

A Guide to Somatic OMing

Check in With Your Body: ... get out of your head, quiet your thoughts, ... and listen for a moment to your body. Feel it. Is it aligned / opposed / confused / resentful ...? To go forward without your body's approval or alignment ... is to invite discord. A big part of OM – for both partners – is developing a stronger *supportive* relationship with our bodies ... and strengthen and develop our intuition (which is just our body's wisdom and voice). And if you lie to your body, overrule it, neglect it ... a lot ... those early check-ins may require you to do a *lot* of damage control – with your relationship with your *own* body. It's part of the practice. You OM better when you are sync with your own body – and it is well nurtured / expressed.

For a stroker, this a more focused instruction. During an OM a coach may remind you to "check in with your body." ... and notice ... "Where does the energy *want* to go?"

Reconnecting to the Body (after an OM): an OM can generate profound altered states ... which can linger and persist after an OM is over. We use 'grounding' techniques at the end of an OM ... to help the strokee 'reconnect to her body.' (See the term "Grounding" above.)

Really ... what grounding means ... is moving her body into a more traditional / 'normal' ... altered state. All conscious states ... are 'altered.' We only agree to pretend a handful of them are "normal." This is illustrated best ... when a person from an aboriginal culture ... "enters" our culture – the jarring part of their experience ... is part of the process of learning a "new normal" – a new baseline for ordinary day-to-day consciousness.

No Eye-Gazing: there are a lot of intimacy practices / exercises in the world. 'Eye-Gazing' is one of them. It's a fine exercise ... but it has no place in OM.

Once the OM begins ... both partners are instructed to focus on the point of connection: the point where the stroker's finger makes contact with the strokee's clit. Some new strokers find themselves succumbing to old conditioning ... and looking to make eye contact with their partner for feedback or approval ... and their strokee will often remind them ... "Hey ... eyes on the / my pussy!" The pussy ... its color shifts, engorgement, and visible twitches and contractions ... are a stroker's best guide to how they are doing in an OM. Women often have been conditioned to lie about feeling pleasure ... in order to receive approval or appear compliant.

The pussy never lies.

No Horsetrading: this a simpler reminder that OM is a 'no-commerce' model. It's a reminder to not get hooked into ... OMing in exchange for *anything.* Even married couples can fall into this trap: "I'll do dishes if we can OM later." A woman should be able to ask for an OM ... without bartering for a blowjob or a new set of Tupperware. Her sex deserves more respect.

It is a privilege and honor to stroke a woman's pussy. Find someone who who can align with that ... and train them how to stroke you. (Or send them to get reputable OM training or coaching.)

(See the entry above for **"No-Commerce" Model.**)

No "Owe-sies:" same as No Horsetrading (see above). A woman does not "owe" her stroker *anything* for OMing with her. No makeouts, no sex, not "just a lil kiss," and not that post-OM hug. Women ... stand up for your pussies.

Place Your Full Attention on Her / Your Clit: attention is a powerful, and – in the west – little understood tool. OM stands for 'Orgasmic Meditation' ... and the meditation part of OM deals with directing our attention in specific ways. One of those ways is to ... "place our full attention on her clit."

In other forms of meditation, there is a phenomena known as "monkey mind." It is the restless, chattering, unsettled, unfocused, and sometimes confused mind. OM is the practice of quieting our monkey mind ... and returning it to the intended focus of our attention: the point of contact of the finger on [one small area of] the clit. As a meditation ... our ability to direct our attention is like a muscle: the more we exercise it, the stronger it becomes.

A Guide to Somatic OMing

The parallel statement ... "place your full attention on her" ... is a reminder ... to use this developing power of focusing our attention ... in our relationships. A woman can tell when we are giving her 20% of our attention. And her pussy keeps track.

Part of honoring a woman is learning to give her your full attention.

Pussy Sensitivity: this is a broad topic. A woman may have a sensitive clitoris ... in general ... or during a specific OM / day. (See the entries for "Stroking the Air Above Her Clit" and "Shards of Glass Sensation.") If she still wants to OM, expect light strokes will be a necessity.

A woman may also have a sensitivity to the material of your gloves. (For more info see here.) She may be sensitive to one of the lube ingredients. (For more info see here.) Her pussy sensitivity may also be due to her period cycle.

  "Stroke the Air Above the Clit:" if you stroke women long enough, eventually you may reach a point one day where she keeps asking you to "go / stroke lighter!" ... repeating the same request until ... suddenly ... you find yourself stroking the air *above* her clit! And she is still connected ... and responding ... to the "air strokes."

It's a real thing. OM is fundamentally an energy-based practice. Although it may take some time before a practitioner begins to grasp that fact experientially. And for most strokers ... the first experience "stroking the air above a woman's clit" ... is their introduction. (See the post on this topic here for more info.)

  "Breathe Through Your Pussy:" this guidance was most often given (in my experience) by women coaching women in our group OMs. This is an advanced adjustment only veteran strokers (in this case, 500+ OMs) should consider giving to their partner. It is almost impossible to language just 'when' it is needed. If you aren't certain, don't use it. There is a limbic correlate that women seem to find ... that has this "make sense" to them. The stroker should not push it. Make the suggestion once ... and then back off. Advanced strokers (1000+) will have a more intuitive read on when to use this. Follow up on your intuition by checking in with her after the OM is complete (after the exchange of frames). Checking and calibrating your intuitions will make you a better stroker – just keep in mind that she *owes* you nothing, including this check-in. (She may not be in a place post-OM for "extra" communications.)

Pushing Out: this is a somatic instruction given to women … it means they should "push out" [energy] through their pussy. Doing so can sometimes free up the flow of energy / orgasm in their system. It won't make much sense to strokers. Once women 'get' it … their bodies can make the adjustment needed. Strokers: if you aren't certain about it, don't use it.

Shards-of-Glass: this is an odd phenomena that about 1/3 of new women OMers go through. They will describe a painful sensation coming from their pussy during an OM when stroked … often using the same phrase … "it feels like shards of glass in my pussy!" There doesn't appear to be any damage or injury to the pussy. It appears as if dormant nerve connections are waking up – kind of like when a foot falls asleep, but *much* more painful. In the 50 or so cases I was around, the women were encouraged to 'OM through it.' And in every case that I know of … it passed … after a few days or weeks.

A woman should always set her own course with her body … and *never* be coached to move through pain in her pussy. And, in fairness, the women who led the Warehouse … would simply tell women what they knew about the sensation … and let them decide for themselves. I heard of no women opting out. All moved forward … and in all cases (that I know of) the sensation went away.

(Note … do not confuse this with your stroker getting sand or some other irritant – or in your pussy – or the lube. Or a crease in glove on the stroking finger can be an irritant as well.)

Locked Hips: sometimes a woman … new to OM … or in a state of high arousal will 'lock' their hips – hold them motionless. Sometimes this happens because the woman unconsciously doesn't want a sensation to end. Other times it is because she is afraid (again unconsciously) that if she even moves … a very tenuous connection may be lost. Yet other times she has been taught to "lay still" and be compliant.

In live OM coaching, a veteran woman OMer (an informal coach) would circulate in a class or circle (with the express consent of the OMers present) … and would often spot a new woman OMer who was 'locking her hips' … and the female coach would gently say … "unlock your hips." And generally … that was all it took. (BTW, the most heard counsel to women in these teaching situations … was "Breathe!" Even experienced strokers would offer this … if they noticed their partner had stopped breathing.)

Relax Your Hips: this is an instruction / reminder to a strokee … to relax (unlock) her hips. Often during an OM … a woman may unconsciously hold their breath or 'lock' their hips … for fear of disrupting an experience …… or in an attempt to 'control' or 'steer' or hold onto it. She has a partner … her stroker … she can (now) afford to relax and let the energy flow.

She doesn't have to do everything herself.

Hip Movement: When some new women begin to OM, their hips move – sometimes a lot. Often this can be traced to the women wanting – consciously or unconsciously – to "help" their stroker … find the 'right spot.' Hip movement is considered 'extra' … and – while it is not bad or wrong – strokees are encouraged to relax their hips and request adjustments of their stroker … when they notice a change their body wants. Partly this is training to ask for what they want … and partly this is to allow the woman to sink even deeper into her involuntary (her limbic system). The [meta] point of OM is to allow a woman to let go completely … and enjoy her own body's sensations.

Body rocking: this is where a strokee is unwilling to ask for the stoke she wants, so she creates it herself … which means she is masturbating, not OMing. Some body rocking is common with some women new to OM. It's just a phase. It can take a while for a woman to adjust … to asking for the stroke she wants – and having that request actually met.

A Guide to Somatic OMing

Keep Track of Your Lube: pristine hygiene in OMs is extremely important: clean OM towels, clean lube, clean gloves ... helps keep a pussy healthy. One of the bad habits new people get into is loaning their lube out to people / strangers. Contaminated lube can lead to painful UTIs (urinary tract infections).

Avoid giving your lube jar to someone who may (through inexperience or carelessness) allow your lube to become contaminated.

If you are at an OM Circle and want to give lube to someone, use a *gloved* hand ... dip into your lube jar ... and transfer a healthy dollop onto a clean unused glove. The stroker can then (carefully) stage the glove with the lube next to them in their nest.

Double-Dipping [into the Lube Supply]: ... is the *very bad* habit of dipping a gloved finger – that has already made contact with her pussy and its fluids (and bacteria) – back into the lube jar (or supply). Basically, you are contaminating the OM lube source (whether it is yours or hers). Close the lid and the next time you OM with it ... surprise!! UTI.

The need for more lube is common in 2 instances: with strokers new to OM; and when starting with a new female partner (she may be drier than you are used to).

The fix is to stash a dollop of lube on a back-up location, for easy reloading. This is often the back of your left glove (unless it is warm ... in which case it will likely slide off). Alternatively, place an extra clean glove within easy reach ... and put the backup dollop on that.

UTIs (urinary tract infections) are a pain for women to deal with. Women who get them will need to give their pussies a rest. OMing [with gloves] is an extremely hygienic practice. Done right ... it is safer than sex.

A Guide to Somatic OMing

OMer's Leg: this is also sometimes called "dead leg" and refers to the right leg of a stroker not getting sufficient circulation ... and becoming numb or sore during an OM. The cause is most frequently insufficient or incorrect support / padding under the stroker's butt and leg(s). Improper seating / support / positioning of the stroker ... can put a strain on their back and muscles and unnecessarily distract them from putting their full attention on stroking their partner. It should be addressed. (Every stroker should stretch and / or do yoga regularly. Even if you are limber now, everyone ages.)

The remedy is to take some time ... when an OM *isn't* taking place ... and experiment (over a fake nest) with firmer (or fluffier) cushions under the right knee ... and possibly raising the stroker's butt with some firm cushions (thereby changing the resting angle of the right hip during the OM). Once the stroker figures out what support they need ... they will be better able to find the right support materials in the next OM.

Also, you may need more pillows / cushions than other OMers. That's fine. Figure out what your body needs and see that it gets the support it requires. (If you travel for OMs, you may need to bring a personal cushion or zafu cushion to guarantee that you meet your needs.)

Pulling for Attention: this is when someone "wants" more attention / intimacy ... and does subtle little manipulations ... to draw you into "spontaneously" offering them what they want. The manipulations in and around an OM Nest are usually for container breaks ... hugs, kisses, a "backrub" etc. The typical ploys may include ... heavily sexualized frames, puppy dog eyes, describing the woman's pussy "as gorgeous," flattery or fawning attention, watching her face "longingly" during the OM. (More can be found in the entry for "Leaking Energy.")

This is a bad habit that most men in the west learn early. Guys who pull for attention will need re-training. If you encounter someone who does this … consider whether you want to re-train them … or direct them elsewhere [for training]. Do they take adjustments well? Or do they quickly / sneakily revert to old habits?

Overstroking: like many OM terms, this has a practical meaning in OM, and is also used metaphorically in everyday life.

When a stroker strokes a clit … particularly if they are a male and are new … they have a tendency to "overstroke." They literally are stroking too much … too fast / too hard. The strokee often reports on their end … a physical irritation or rising sensitivity and / or a sense of disconnection from their stroker. Overstroking happens with newbies. It is a calibration thing … that's all. Most people … in their ordinary lives … have never stroked a point so small on a surface so sensitive … with such deliberateness. It's as if when new strokers start, they are OMing with mittens on. The most frequent adjustments a new stroker is likely to receive is … "lighter…" and "slower…."

In the outside world, when someone is talking too much or has made their point … and is *still* talking … we say they are overstroking. It is a useful shorthand. Even with oneself. Many OMers – men and women – catch themselves 'over-explaining' … and simply remind themselves, "I'm overstroking." The adjustment often happens automatically.

After all, no one likes a sore clit.

Dumping On: this is when one person 'uses' a second person (often without consent or safeporting) … to "dump" their problems / energy / woes / complaints onto. This can often lead to the second person "blowing out" (see term above).

By way of contrast, in a consensual context, the second person can act as a terminal to "ground" some the excess energy. They provide – willingly – very valuable support.

A Guide to Somatic OMing

In a nonconsensual context, the same thing occurs. Only, instead of partnering with the second person ... the "dumper" just flat out *uses* them ... ignoring their partner's humanity / needs.

This relates to OM ... because tumesced people often need to "discharge" some of their excess energies. They can "dump" on someone ... or they can OM with someone. OM is a great reliever – for both strokee and stroker – of built up energy / tumescence.

Over-OMing: this is a real thing, although denied by OM trainers for years. Humans share a common physiology ... with individuals falling in different places at different times ... with respect to what is considered 'normal' ... biologically-speaking. So ...

... One: OMing depends on adequate grounding to not leave its practitioners in an unstable 'high' state. And grounding has been a weak afterthought for much of the existence of OM. It was much more fun to reach ecstatic highs – and the OM culture bestowed a 'coolness' status on that – than do the more mundane 'come-down' stage of grounding. As of the date of this writing, most OMers do a less-than-adequate job of grounding *either* the strokee or the stroker. Which means that for some OMers who OM a lot ... and don't ground enough ... they can be said to be "over-OMing." Basically, the body needs to complete certain cycles ... in order to maintain a healthy equilibrium. Inadequate grounding can have an impact on the body. [...] So this example may be less a case of over-OMing and more a case of a sloppy or incomplete practice.

... Two: more seriously, some people's hormonal systems and / or nervous systems are already in or close to the red ... before they ever start to OM. OM can have a powerful impact on the hormonal and nervous systems. And for people in or close to the red neurotically ... the impact of OMing regularly can be strikingly different ... than it is for most people.

... Three: OMing churns up a *lot* of psychological stuff that may previously have been unconsciousness. For some people, that's a good thing. For others ... notsomuch. It can be annoying, destabilizing, or worse. If you get overwhelmed, stop. Take a break. Or discontinue the practice entirely. Not everyone likes bungiejumping. Find an activity that suits you and supports you in the way you want / need to be supported.

If you are having unusual physical reactions to OMing, stop OMing and check with your physician. OMing is a sex act ... and while it is unlikely to cause any more biological impact than regular [protected] sex, unusual reactions may signal body imbalances (for example, in hormonal or nervous systems) that were previously hidden or unnoticed. Get them checked out.

And if anyone tells you ... "you just need to OM more!!" ... feel free to tell them OM is a practice – not a cult.

And listen to your body.

Taking a Break [from OMing]: during the Warehouse era, the coaching was often "just OM more!" ... when any concern, issue, or obstacle arose. We were an experimental community.

But that blanket guidance is reckless and irresponsible for anybody who is a part of the real world.

There are any number of reasons to take a break from – or stop entirely – an intense somatic practice.

- ✦ because you feel like it;
- ✦ because you have a UTI;
- ✦ you can't currently process the personal issues it is bringing up;
- ✦ it's too much work;
- ✦ nothing is happening;
- ✦ you're bored;

- ◆ you have finished an incredibly productive cycle and want to digest it;
- ◆ you are stretched too thin in your existing commitments;
- ◆ no reliable, trained partners are available;
- ◆ you don't feel safe;
- ◆ you want more training and / or support;
- ◆ the local politics are too filled with drama / angst / instability;
- ◆ to check out it feels to *not* OM for a while.;
- ◆ for no particular reason.

OM is not a cult. It is a practice. Make sure it is working for you … or set it aside.

The world is a large, rich, diverse, mysterious, wondrous place. Be curious.

* * *

Stroking

Bread and Butter Stroke: the simplest, basic stroke (medium pressure, speed, length) in an OM. The first stroke most OMers learn (after the lube stroke).

Lube Stroke: this is the first stroke in the OM. It distributes the lube where it is needed (the clit) … while keeping it away from areas where it is not needed (the clitoral hood). Getting lube on the hood makes it almost impossible to (gently) pull the hood back with the gloved left thumb … it becomes too slippery. (Complete instructions can be found in the 2017 OT Container doc.)

Upstroke: in OM the stroker strokes the woman's clit … in a light up-and-down motion. Upstrokes are lighter and faster strokes … with just the very tip of the stroking finger. Upstrokes bring the woman's energy up. Upstrokes are often described as having airy, ethereal, soaring energy.

At a slightly more complex level, the [experienced] stroker can 'intend' either 'up' or 'down' … irrespective of the actual physical direction of the stroke. This is a part of the energy aspect of OM.

In a typical OM cycle (lasting seconds or minutes), a stroker brings their partner's energy up … until it flips and wants to go 'down.' Then the stroker takes the energy 'down.' When it goes 'down' far enough … the energy flips again and wants to go 'up.' The stroker's instructions are … to 'feel' the shift (flip) coming … and change direction right *before* the energy shifts. This preserves some of the energy … and speeds the build up of energy / orgasm.

Upstrokes are not *better* than downstrokes. Both are needed in an OM. Some people have a natural preference for upstrokes or downstrokes (generally the ratio is about 4 : 1 … up : down). And some people will go through phases where their body craves one or the other.

Outside of an OM … 'upstrokes' are a metaphor for any communication / action / interaction … that brings a person 'up' energetically or emotionally. Upstrokes can include compliments, praise, approval, and acknowledgements. Again … upstrokes are not 'better' than downstrokes We need both downstrokes and upstrokes … to have a full, rounded experience of life.

Downstroke: when the clit is stroked in an OM, the basic movement of the stroking finger is up-down, up-down. A downstroke is firmer and slower … done with broad, meaty strokes … using the whole pad of the finger, instead of just the tip. Downstrokes bring the woman's energy down. Downstrokes are often described as having earthy, 'fucking,' grounding energy.

At a slightly more complex level, the [experienced] stroker can 'intend' either 'up' or 'down' … irrespective of the actual physical direction of the stroke. This is a part of the energy aspect of OM.

A Guide to Somatic OMing

In a typical OM cycle (lasting seconds or minutes), a stroker brings their partner's energy up … until it flips and starts to go 'down.' Then the stroker takes the energy 'down.' When it goes 'down' far enough … the energy flips again and starts to go 'up.' The stroker's instructions are … to 'feel' the shift (flip) coming … and change direction right *before* the energy shifts. This preserves some of the energy (momentum) … and speeds the build up of energy / orgasm.

Upstrokes are not *better* than downstrokes. Both are needed in an OM. Some people have a natural preference for upstrokes or downstrokes (generally the ratio is about 4 : 1 … up : down). And some people will go through phases where their body craves one or the other.

Outside of an OM … 'downstrokes' are a metaphor for any communication / action / interaction … that brings a person 'down' energetically or emotionally. Examples can include blunt criticism or bad news. "That was quite a downstroke." Again … downstrokes are not 'bad.' We need both downstrokes and upstrokes … to have a full, rounded experience of life.

Resonant Stroke: in the mythos of OM … a 'resonant stroke' … is an especially sweet or deeply nourishing stroke. The best analogy I have … is you when you have an itch … and someone is scratching your back. Their scratching can feel "kinda" good … as they zero in on the itch. But when they hit "the spot" – it feels *a-maz-ing.* So too in OM … your stroker can be stroking you … you can be feeling pleasure … and then suddenly your stroker – consciously or unconsciously – makes a small adjustment … AND … OH … MY … GAWD! It isn't just pleasurable – it resonates with your body in a way you didn't know you wanted. That's an example of a 'resonant stroke.'

[a] **Light Stroke:** 2 uses. The first use is in OM: an actual light stroke on the clitoris by the stroker. Generally, when new strokers learn to OM … they stroke too heavily. (See the entry "Stroking the Air Above Her Clit.") The antidote – and the coaching – is frequently "use a lighter stroke."

The second use is as a metaphor in general communications. Again … "light stroke" implies that many of our communications are too heavy, too ponderous, too wordy ... and could be "lightened up."

So ... in both cases, you will hear, "Remember ... [use] a light stroke."

* * *

:: Energy Patterns & Cycles ::

Apotheosis: this is a state a woman can encounter in an OM where ... everything stops, she becomes completely still. There is often a feeling of timelessness. She's may not be doing contractions anymore, her hands may be frozen open and she may look almost like a statue, but her stroker can feel tremendous surges of energy going through her body, but the surges of energy aren't going out of her body, they are going in. (Note that apotheosis is not a goal in OM ... just a really cool state one can encounter.)

The word 'apotheosis' is_ taken from the Greek, meaning "glorification to a divine level" or "to deify" or "becoming god-like." It is a state reached in orgasmic meditation experienced as both an expansion in consciousness where a person transcends binary existence, and a pure, locked sensation of the most still, peaceful and absorbing silence. In this state a person may feel completely nourished, hydrated and fulfilled. (Wikipedia :: https://en.wikipedia.org/wiki/Apotheosis)

The general guidance to a stroker if their partner seems to be 'in' this state is ... don't change anything and don't try to "steer" or direct this. Just wait it out ... and let your partner have her ride. Quiet your energy ... ("I am a leaf on the wind.") Afterwards, finish the OM ... and check in with her after the OM is complete (including exchanging frames).

Being "Held" (not the 'hugs' kind): This kind of 'held' is nonsexual and gender-neutral. It means to 'hold space for someone' ... so they can undergo a potentially cathartic set of experiences. It means you have their back. You won't creep on them, 'hit' on them, or otherwise take advantage of them ... while their full attention is elsewhere. A physical correlate for 'being held' is partnered rope climbing – when you are 'on belay' ... your partner is "literally" *holding you ... on the "safety" [belay] rope. And they have their *full* attention on you and on keeping you safe ... while you explore new rock surfaces / heights.

Part of 'being held' for OMers is being well-trained in what OM is – and what it isn't. (It isn't an opportunity to 'hit on' or grope someone ... and is *not* foreplay, for some examples). And part is being clear and clean in your communications ... and checking with your partner when new terrain is encountered. And part is being mindful of – and fully responsible for – your right range.

Being [Fully] Met: means showing up in a skillful, powerful, authentic, truthful way ... in support of your partner. You show up – fully ... and they show up – fully.

Being Seen: is the act of energetically witnessing someone. This often happens when someone reveals something vulnerable and / or authentic ... and observes that another person was watching / listening ... and actually *noticed* the deeply personal share – and did not turn away / deflect it. It is a form of intimate connection ... and is deeply nourishing in a specific way ... a way that the body recognizes. People who don't have (or don't track very well) a sense of "being seen" often act out, are disruptive, or are needy for attention. It takes skill and awareness ... to notice when you are being "seen." Some people are often ignored ... while others are seen ... but can't track that.

Blowing Out [a Stroker]: to 'blow someone out' means that they are overwhelmed with energy or charge ... and, as a result, they are only partially present / functional.

A Guide to Somatic OMing

In particularly high or energetic OMs ... a stroker – after the OM – may be "blown out." This isn't a bad thing, per se. It is kind of like going on a very intense roller coaster. They will need some time to reboot (or 'come down') ... before they can interact effectively. Being 'blown out' is an extreme case of ungroundedness.

As usual, the OM concept transfers nicely ... to ordinary life. An argument – or an unexpected party – can "blow someone out," as well. Same principle.

Depletion: A person may become depleted energetically. Being depleted weakens one's ability to be present, hold energy in an OM, and make good decisions generally.

While learning to OM and starting a practice can take a lot of energy initially, the practice in the long run can be extremely nourishing energetically to women ... and even to their strokers. This process is called 'filling up'* and it is the antithesis of being depleted. (*There are other activities which 'fill' a person up ... in slightly different ways ... like hiking, dancing, creating art.)

Desire: desire is a central concept / experience in OM. Desire arises in the body. You may imagine skydiving in your mind ... but until it lands (shows up) in your body as a rise in excitement (desire), it is just an 'idea.' OM teaches us how to connect – be present to – our desires as they arise in our body. Many people who begin to OM have desire and anxiety deeply conflated ... to the point where they just register 'numbness' to get some relief. OMing gradually teaches them that it is okay to actually *feel* desires ... and feeling them is distinct and different from acting on them.

The OM practice also helps us separate desire ... from request. In western culture, desire and request are often collapsed, so that a person stating a desire ... is heard by another person ... as making an imaginary request. (See also the FB Note on "Distinction Between Desire & Request.")

Expansion: An expansion is an increase or rise in the energy [in a person]. A person bursting into laughter can be said to be expanding [energetically] ...

while if they stop suddenly when a teacher enters the room, they can be said to be contracting [energetically]. Energy – whether in a room, an individual, a conversation, or an OM – ebbs and flows constantly. It rarely stays at the same level in nature. The 'ebbs' are contractions, the 'flows' are expansions. This can be applied to communities as well as individuals. An OM community can be said to be 'expanding' (growing) or 'contracting' (shrinking).

Filling Up: This is a complex term, with many levels. At its most basic level, an OM is designed to support women in "filling up" ... with a much needed type of energetic nourishment: sensual limbic connection with another human being ... with that person's full attention, and with unconditional approval. The state of culture in the west is such that ... most women are not touched *with approval* enough, their sex is often rudely dismissed as secondary in importance to men's orgasm and pleasure, and their partners rarely give the woman's sex their full undivided attention. As a result, most women are "parched" somatically ... and get by with their "connection" well or tank ... dangerously low or empty. The practice of OM allows women to "get filled up" and become "hydrated."

It can take 2 years or more for a woman with an 'active' OM practice (12+ OMs per week) ... to get "filled up." And that state ... being "filled up" ... is a very definite state or somatic address. Women who reach it ... report noticing that their body has shifted ... that their bodies are no longer running checks in the background ... wondering where the next 'fix' of limbic intimacy is going to come from. They can feel their bodies relax ... and open up. Their field of awareness becomes much larger ... and they often experience a [new] feeling of curiosity about their world.

Men who stroke women ... are nourished as well ... through being in the field of a woman's orgasm regularly. They may experience a different kind of "filling up." The disparity of what men can get and what women are 'allowed' in the west ... is huge, however. There are other practices that can address men's other energetic or limbic needs. OM is designed to address and correct a cultural imbalance (and deficit) most women experience – and have had to put up with.

A Guide to Somatic OMing

OM is designed – and reserved specifically – for … helping end the cultural drought … for limbic connection in women's lives. A woman has the inalienable right to ask for an OM … be stroked … and then get up and go about her day … owing her partner *nothing.*

Full (2 uses): In OM there are two common uses of "full" … both distinctly different.

The first use is related to the concept of "filling up." At its most basic level, an OM is designed to support women in "filling up" … with a much needed type of energetic nourishment: sensual limbic connection with another human being … with that person's full attention, and with unconditional approval.

The second use of "I'm full" comes in conversation … or in the course of listening to a lengthy explanation (say, about OM). Basically, there may come a point where "your ears are full" … and even if they keep talking … nothing more is going in. Among [some] OMers … we give ourselves permission to say in such instances, "I'm full." The courteous / prudent response is … to stop talking immediately (if it is just the 2 of you). After all, the glazed look in their eyes usually confirms … nothing more will go in. They need a break. If, however, the speaker chooses *not* to stop talking … well, in OM we would call that "overstroking" – stroking past the point of pleasure. It is a newbie mistake.

It is explained in detail here … https://www.facebook.com/theOMreport/posts/996869707067434

Tumescence: in OM tumescence is considered unutilized or potential energy. When we're in approval — when we're in flow with our life and our surroundings — this energy fuels turn-on / orgasm. If we are tense or clenched or blocked in some way, tumescence can manifest as irritation and bodily discomfort. Tumescent energy is most pleasurably experienced when it is well-utilized, not sitting idle. Energy wants to flow.

Ungrounded: in an OM if someone is still 'high' after the OM ... they are ungrounded. (See the term "Grounding" above.) (For more info on OM grounding tips, see here.)

Note that once you get the concept ... you will notice out in the 'real world' ... when ordinary people are "ungrounded." And yes, regular grounding advice might be helpful to them. Proceed with caution. Be mindful of social boundaries, informed consent, and ordinary decorum.

Poor Grounding: if someone is 'high' or spacey after an OM, it is usually due to inadequate grounding. Unfortunately, many traditional OM teachers have said that only a few minutes of grounding are necessary ... and implicitly ... that 'women need to toughen up or get with the program.'

That's cynical marketing talking ... not wisdom. Many women's needs will fluctuate greatly from OM to OM. Strokers should learn to recognize the signs of "may-need-more-grounding" ... and partners should schedule a 'more grounding' time cushion into their OM appointments ... just in case. Also, OM Circles should provide a final grounding time buffer after the last OM round ... and not have to chase people out before they are sufficiently grounded.

Leaking Energy: this is common when someone is unconsciously – or even consciously but covertly – "pulling" [silently] for an outcome. This is often represented for people ... when they sense a divergent outcome at play – a person X may say one thing, but seems to want something opposite. One example is when an OM is complete and the stroker is about to depart ... one person may seem to 'want' a hug – even though they have an agreement 'not' to hug after OMs. Calling it 'leaking energy' allows one to keep their observation neutral – and avoid being reactive or accusatory. It allows a simple check-in to take place: "I'm sensing an energy leak from you. Do you desire [x] right now? Consistent with the separation of Desire & Request ... their companion (the energy leaker) ... is free to check their body and answer truthfully – knowing that stating a desire they have in their body ... is not an actual request. "Yeah ... I do notice a desire for a hug right now." "Cool. Thanks."

A Guide to Somatic OMing

In that example, a person was able to notice in their body that something was 'off' in the other person ... do a quick clean check-in ... get confirmation of their 'read' ... and go about their day. No upset ... mystery cleared up ... boundaries & agreements maintained. (For more on **Distinguishing Desire & Request** see this FB Note.)

Dissipate the Energy (*e.g.*, thru nervous chatter): one of the first lessons I learned when I started OMing ... was to become conscious when energy was being [unwittingly] dissipated. In a conversation, one party may break eye contact ... or laugh nervously ... or make a joke. All are ways we use to drop the energy / sensation in our body ... when we are feeling "too much." (Most OM lessons transfer nicely to the context of having conversations with people.)

In OM we are concentrating on building energy up ... and being able to 'hold' more energy. (I know ... it's a goalless practice. But this is how it plays out. And yes ... it's still a goalless practice.) Every time a woman "goes over" (climaxes) in an OM, her energy drops and she has to start over. It is a lot like surfing. I can paddle a short way out ... catch a small wave ... ride it for a few seconds. And then my ride is over. And I have to paddle back out. Or I paddle for a longer time ... catch a big wave ... and have a *much* longer ride. Climax is equivalent to the wipeout at the end of riding the wave.

The more experienced women OMers figure this out – whether they have been taught this or not. They discover they like "riding the wave of orgasm" during an OM. And when they climax / go over ... they find they have to start over (paddle back out) ... building up energy. The sweet spot ... is riding the wave – and just like surfers – and avoid wiping out as long as they can. Experienced women – and some newbies – can start an OM already in high state of turn-on / orgasm (e.g., their pussy is already contracting) ... and they just intensify that orgasm throughout the OM ... and ride that ever-increasing wave of orgasm – without going over – for the *whole OM.*

A Guide to Somatic OMing

Dissipating energy is what you do when you don't know what to do with the energy ... or you can't *hold* (feel the energy and stay conscious / present) very much energy ... without blowing out. It is a form of unintended self-grounding.

* * *

PART 2

THE MISSING 10% ::

I mentioned in the Introduction that I realized during the Warehouse era that we came 90% of the way to developing a full, clean code version of OM. That fully-realized vision of OM would allow people to make some exceptional leaps in training and human development. I have long range plans that hinge on being able to leverage a virus-free pool of experienced OMers. Those plans require that *someone* cough up a clean code version of OM ... complete with that missing 10%.

What is a 'Clean Code' Version of OM? ::

A 'clean code' version of OM is a public model of OM free of somatic malware or viruses. Somatic malware and viruses are instructions that undermine or are at odds with the central design and intent of OM: to source and support empowering women around their sexuality, orgasm, expression, agency, and voice. The core model of OM *is* relatively clean. But *how* people have often been introduced to OM via a sales culture ... often introduces 'bad code' (e.g., "unleash your beast mode," FOMO, etc.) which is often conflated with – and mistaken for – OM culture. As a result, what people 'think' is OM ... and what actually constitutes OM ... is sometimes vastly different.

Generating a public 'clean code' version / model of OM is a key step in creating a safer practice and a safer OM community.

What is 'the Missing 10%'? ::

Classic OM needs some additional pieces and some refinements ... if it is going reach the potential I see for it. To close the remaining gap, I need a few additions, upgrades, and modifications made to the Classic Model of OM.

A Guide to Somatic OMing

In addition to simply cleanly separating a *public* model of OM from all the failed experimental modifications and extensions (Sex Magic?!) that have accrued over the years, we need clarification and expansion of the connection between OM and truthtelling. Commercial interests have fogged / muddied / compromised the connection and seriously impacted the somatic maps people [OMers] built of OM.

We need a more robust Soma Model ... one that expands and builds on the Pussy-Centric Model. While the connection to – and concept of – the soma is deeply embedded in learning to OM and the practice itself, our genitals are not the sole basis of our existence and choices. We can go deeper.

We need a model of cultures ... that can serve as a value-neutral bridge for OM discoveries. We need fewer pushy 'OM evangelicals' evangelizing ... and more seasoned OMers quietly contributing to other cultures "as-they-are." We need to reach out and contribute to non-OMers ... not coax, seduce, and trick them. (Again, some of these are concerns about the sales culture ... which has become conflated with OM culture).

We need better skills bank design overall and better support for community-level training, expression, leadership, and agency. Historically, OM rising stars have been undermined and sidelined, leaving the OM community with a deficit of strong, independent leaders. We especially need better support for women's training, expression, leadership, and agency.

We need more and better designs ... for ritualized communications ... to convey increasing esoteric (by mainstream culture's standards) experiences and somatic references. We have a lot to communicate, and we are better off when we can communicate efficiently and with precision. (The distinctions that the soma makes available will be key.)

We need better training and support for distinguishing and responsibly managing trauma-related incidents, both old triggered instances of PTSD as well as fresh traumas. OM stirs a *lot* up, often very quickly. OM has been to date ... a mostly "sink-or-swim" culture with respect to trauma. This needs to change.

We need better and more sophisticated training and support for failure recovery and error correction, particularly for male OMers. Mainstream culture has taught them ... poorly. They typically come to OM with skewed understandings of agency – both theirs and women's – and often have gaslighting, bullying ("dominating"), and deflection ... as perfectly acceptable communication options – for them. OM can offer a structured environment to retrain and 'recover' men ... into a more equitable social dynamic.

We need to retire the 'sink-or-swim' model of OM training in favor of graduated pipelines to OMing ... with heavy emphasis on graduated prerequisites to How to OM. This will generate less trauma ... and more nuanced discovery. We need to create, refine, and make available ... flexible OM 'prep' courses ... to ease the experience of learning ... How to OM. OM culture is deep and often intense. Instead of tossing newbies in the deep end of the pool, we can distinguish and offer a series of OM Prep (preparation) courses and training options. Part of the reason my experience of OM was so rich was I built up knowledge which supported my OM practice through the course of taking a number of weekend-long OM-related classes. Some of these new OM Prep courses might be: Orientation to Women's Social Experiences (for Men); Communication Basics 101, Orientation to the Pussy (separate Courses for Men & Women); and Ethics, Agency, & Consent. Many of these OM Prep courses could be available online (and free with no 'sign-up' required) for easy review and (re)familiarization. It is unwise and a disservice to simply 'dump' new people interested in OM directly into truncated 'How to OM' courses.

We need creation and promotion of better feedback channels and communication rituals … to OM communities and instructors (and coaches) for OM courses / training. We especially need to eliminate any support or tolerance for gaslighting and the hoarding of information related to the safe practice of OM.

We need to strongly discourage the treatment by OM-related businesses of OMers (and people who are new-to-OM) as primarily "potential sales prospects." That scarcity mentality is in opposition to the core tenets of OM. Same with sales people creating and leveraging FOMO (Fear Of Missing Out). Few things have been as corrosive long term to the flourishing of OM and OMers as this particular predatory sales gimmick.

We need to build and make available training for converting complaints and concerns into actionable positive steps or 'suggested' standards. This is an important dimension of personal agency. At the same time, groups, communities, and organizations should not be let off the hook … by insisting that people who identify breakdowns or failings in a community … be obligated to "find the fix" themselves. This is an important dimension of tribal or group agency. If the complainer hasn't the skills or bandwidth currently … to parse their core complaint into an actionable 'fix,' it is on the group – and the group's leaders – to close that gap. No more hiding from group agency … by hiding behind a facade of 'respect' for personal agency.

We need to surface and have frank conversations about the vetting / screening / gatekeeping processes in OM communities, as well as those by individuals. Safety matters. Identifying and publicizing both the Best Practices and Worst Practices will be an important step forward.

We need to improve and deepen OM's core ethical model … utilizing a differentiated model of personal (and group) agencies. By making agency training explicit and recognized … we can assist OMers in better translating their OM expertise into non-OM (and G-rated) contexts. A vast amount of early OM experience for new OMers is simply making adjustments to their gendered models of agency – who can and can't do (or say) what.

We need to [formally] introduce the principle of arousal nonconcordance (the concept that agency arises in the *whole* soma ... not just in the signals / sensations in the genitals). Aspects of this are implicit in the distinction between Desire and Request, but not a lot of OMers have that training ... or distinction.

Finally, we need to shift in the long term ... the ultimate arbitrar / authority of 'what is OM' to the OM community or an independent body ... not a private corporation.

* * *

A Guide to Somatic OMing

INTRODUCING SOMATIC OMING ::

Somatic OMing represents the deeper practice that I have encountered during my OMing practice.

Somatic OMing is based on the Classic Model of OM. It focuses on using OMing to foster and develop ... energy skills and awareness; enhanced ability around truthtelling; a deeper relationship with one's own soma ... and the soma of others; the ability to work more effectively on teams and in groups; and the ability to create, modify, and troubleshoot sound, ethical social games.

Somatic OMing is a reference frame / model ... designed to operate *around* a Classic OM practice. It is a way of organizing and elevating / fine-tuning some of the experiences of traditional OMing ... in order to strengthen and deepen intuition and intuitive processes and develop other underdeveloped aspects of 'being human:' identity, truthtelling, game design (and 'play'), agency, mastery, storytelling, expression, integrity.

*   *   *

At its most basic Somatic OMing is about becoming adept at telling the truth, working more fluidly in community, cleaning out the soma, and becoming highly skilled with energy [numina].

A Guide to Somatic OMing

Most seasoned OMers know that OMing is messy ... it isn't all sparky highs and erotic arcs. Intense emotions like sadness, grief, rage, and confusion often arise in OMs. Many new OMers – strokers and strokees alike – report numbness or no sensation at all ... often for their first 50 OMs or more. Gradually the connection to the soma / body (re)awakens ... and some of the most valued OM experiences revolve around authenticity, [deep] resonance, and simple connection. This is the realm of Somatic OMing.

* * *

A Guide to Somatic OMing

AN ANALYSIS OF SOMATIC OMING CULTURE ::

The section on cultural analysis lays out a methodology for analyzing cultures that was directly and significantly influenced by OM … called The Gaia Vedas (TGV). Aspects of Classic OM are analyzed in light of TGV concepts and principles … deepening the reader's understanding and appreciation of OM's design … and laying out the foundation of Somatic OMing.

* * *

TGV ("The Gaia Vedas") is a system to model and map continuums. It also proves handy, it turns out, when mapping cultures. I use it here to distinguish, illuminate, and map elements of Somatic OM Culture.

There are 12 knowledge domains (called vedas) that will be examined.

- Soma
- Veritas
- Agency
- Games
- Shadow
- Mythos
- Mastery
- Tribe
- Orgasm
- Numina
- Identity
- Planet

* * *

Soma & OM ::

What This Is ...

The soma – or 'body' – is the matrix out of which consciousness arises.

Cortex (or cortex-based) Consciousness is a subset of the much broader Soma Consciousness. Altered states (moods, emotions, 'feelings') – as well as so-called 'normal' states of consciousness – can all be considered somatic addresses ... each representing different, unique 'addresses' that a soma can generate. A single soma – much like a symphony – can generate multiple simultaneous, overlapping somatic addresses (SAs).

How It Connects With Classic OM ...

Classic OM contrasts traditional cortex-based 'knowing' (consciousness) ... with 'limbic' [i.e., somatic] 'knowing' (consciousness).

The OMer expressions ... "the body / pussy knows" ... translates into "the soma knows." A woman who OMs can be said to be rebuilding her relationship with her pussy – or her soma.

OM restores and refreshes / renews our connection to our intuition ... which is a key aspect of soma consciousness.

OM generates a plethora of somatic addresses (altered states) ... many of them new to first-time OMers.

Guidance for Somatic OMing & the Soma ...

All OMs can be considered dialogues with the soma ... one's own soma and the soma of your OM partner.

A Guide to Somatic OMing

The soma is the seat of consciousness.

The soma is the 'source' of intuition. Intuition often needs testing, calibration, and fine-tuning. Some of that happens naturally … some has to be deliberately fostered and engaged in.

Many of our actions arise from (mostly unexamined and / or out-of-date) somatic scripts.

Soma knowledge and skills are a lacking in huge way in most modern / western cultures.

OM allows one to establish or rebuild a relationship and fundamental rapport with their own soma.

OM restores a deeper connection to the soma – both our soma and that of others – and brings established rituals, agreements, and a shared language to the [neglected] domain of the soma.

OM allows practitioners to test, recalibrate, and refine their soma's intuitions and strengthen their existing (or dormant) intuitiveness.

The soma is a central (although unrecognized) aspect of OM. OM fosters a growing intuitive sense and sensibility … which in time comes to represented in some OMers … "my body says ____."

* * *

Veritas & OM ::

What This Is ...

Veritas is about truthtelling.

How It Connects With Classic OM ...

The old SensComm lessons trained OMers in essential communication skills ... including detecting deflections, withholds, deception (lies), and truths.

The practice of OM is the practice of learning to tell the truth again ... to yourself, your soma, your OM partner, and to their soma. You learn to notice and tell the truth about ... what's happening in your soma [body], your desires, requests that do / don't want to make, sensations, emotions, behaviors (blocking / deflecting, lying, withholding, being vulnerable, being present, being 'locked' / frozen). You learn to tell the truth somatically ... by being present, centered, vulnerable, open, connected, curious.

Sharing frames ... trains OMers in one aspect of giving clean reports. Clean reports and communications are tools OMers [can] have ... in cutting down on the crap that clogs up many relationships and communication channels.

Guidance for Somatic OMing & Veritas ...

Make truthtelling a practice.

Own your narrative. Recover personal shadow information and integrate it into an expanded, authentic personal narrative (mythos).

Rebuild / strengthen rapport with your own soma ... and with other somas. A

A Guide to Somatic OMing

lot of unnecessary deception and deflection occurs when people are out of rapport with the soma.

Learn to give – and receive – clean requests and communications … and to make (and maintain) clean agreements.

* * *

Agency & OM ::

What This Is ...

Agency is a dimension of power; it is the ability to act and express oneself.

How It Connects With Classic OM ...

OM restores agency to women that mainstream culture had driven underground, blocked, or made taboo. Men (and other gender expressions) become allies in creating a more equitable, authentic set of social agreements around [personal] agency.

OM is designed to support women's expression, voice, and sexual agency. Through requests for OMs – and for adjustments in an OM – women get to have the OM ... and relationship to orgasm ... they want.

Guidance for Somatic OMing & Agency ...

Much of personal agency arises in the context of community. Learn to make – and receive – clean requests. Learn to make – and keep – clean agreements.

Give the soma a voice ... not only your soma, but all somas you encounter. Most communication is somatic / nonverbal. Dial in. Pay attention. Translate into words when necessary.

Learn to unpack social games ... and distinguish good agency designs ... from poor agency designs. Boundaries are 'real' for [many] people 'playing' in social games.

People will screw up. Develop tribal rituals for failure recovery & error correction. Ostracization is incredibly expensive – and wasteful – to the community. Figure out paths and rituals for people who violate trust /

A Guide to Somatic OMing

boundaries / agreements ... that protect the community ... while offering sensible options for retraining and the renewal / restoration / recovery of social contracts.

* * *

Games & OM ::

What This Is ...

Social Games are the shared imagined constructs we use to create cultures and civilizations.

A fundamental component of human culture is the design, generation, and use of [social] games. A social game is a shared imagined construct ... that we agree to act "as-if" it is real. All social games are founded on a set of agreements ... the 'rules' of the game. The 'boundaries' of the game – together with the rules / agreements of conduct [agency] – are known as the 'game container.'

How It Connects With Classic OM ...

OM is an excellent instance of a created – and well-designed – social game ... which also happens to have deep roots in the soma.

Learning how to OM ... and establishing a strong practice ... can be a Master Class in Game Design.

The OM container is an excellent prototype for designing other social containers.

The instruction set for OM is a classic case of a collection of stories and narratives ... 'inventing' a shared (and imagined) practice. Narratives flourish in community. Squashing or hiding stories from the community ... forces valuable information, energy, resources, and attention ... into the shadow ... to be dealt with / recovered later.

A Guide to Somatic OMing

Guidance for Somatic OMing & Games ...

Use OM as an example ... extract (and test) the tenets of good social game design. Then design other social games: classes, projects, organizations, and group endeavors. (See the section in this book on the Missing 10% ... for insights on filling in design gaps and flaws.)

Make your designs explicit and public ... open to the feedback, criticism, experimentation, testing and input of others.

Create game charter libraries of the best – and worst – social game designs. Turn a list of complaints, problems, or concerns into a 'code of conduct' prototype ... for evaluation and consideration.

* * *

Shadow & OM ::

What This Is ...

The Shadow is whatever information or patterns do not fit with an established or endorsed narrative. It acts as kind of buffer, attic, or [dark] storage for whatever is currently out of fashion.

How It Connects With Classic OM ...

OM surfaces a *lot* of the processes, beliefs, scripts, and choices people are unconscious around ... as well as surfacing 'unowned' desires, actions, tactics, and strategies of theirs.

How they tend to play in social games ... and how they treat [social game] containers ... is often revealed ... through OMing and OM-related interactions.

Much of OM is designed to safely surface and usefully route shadow information ... where it can be processed and reintegrated. Instead of having shadow stuff randomly blowing up.

Guidance for Somatic OMing & the Shadow ...

OM brings up a lot of our crap: name it ... and own it ... while being careful to distinguish between ... desires and requests / requests-for-action. Watch for spikes in the energy. If things get too intense ... you will likely fail ... and to deal with it yet another time. (In OM ... it's called 'blowing out.')

A Guide to Somatic OMing

Owning one's shadow ... is tied directly to learning to tell one's [self the] truth ... and crafting an expanded, empowering, and more complete (and authentic) personal narrative [mythos] ... and can – potentially – simplify and smooth communications and interactions with others.

* * *

Mythos & OM ::

What This Is...

Mythos is the use of stories and narratives to convey instructions.

We order and re-order our worlds through the stories we choose to repeat and give prominence to in our lives. The use of 'story' to order our personal and shared 'worlds' is called mythos. Mythos is also called ... story, narrative, myth, history / histories, bio (biography), science, and religion.

How It Connects With Classic OM ...

OM is a fundamentally different narrative than other mainstream narratives. It is a women-centered narrative, with different values (connection, safe spaces), different distinctions (arousal, energy), and different models of agency (partnerships that honor women's voices and experiences).

OM allows practitioners to deconstruct atrophied or calcified cultural narratives around arousal, agency, status, beauty, desire, orgasm, and the generation of public – and private – avatars. OM allows practitioners to ... over time ... drop into their bodies and experience authentic sensation ... with less out-of-date story encrusted on top.

OM narratives – both first person and historical – disrupt mainstream culture's narratives ... about agency, the body, orgasm, sex, consent, and women ... and men.

OM strives to displace endless recursive, disconnected stories ... for direct experience / sensation and connection to the soma ... separating layers of stories and conflicting narratives from direct experience of 'what's so' ... valuing gnosis over abstracted maps.

A Guide to Somatic OMing

Guidance for Somatic OMing & Mythos ...

Learn to identify, source, and track the stories / narratives that you – and your tribes and communities – are invested in.

Learn to actively craft and shape new narratives ... with new destinations / possibilities and room for new discoveries (edits to the existing mythos).

Learn to identify and become proficient in ... some of the ways we have to convey stories: verbally, somatically, energetically, ritually ... and through urban planning, legislation, architecture, media rules and regulations, 'approved' history books, and 'sanctioned' algorithms.

* * *

Mastery & OM ::

What This Is ...

Mastery is expertise expressed as a dimension of agency.

How It Connects With Classic OM ...

As a community-based practice, most of the 'discovered' maps about OM ... arise organically in community ... among its practitioners. Fostering – or inhibiting – sharing of discoveries and experiences by OM practitioners ... directly impacts the 'wealth' of OM communities.

As a practice, OM is a perfect lab / reference for exploring the arc of mastery ... and how access to mastery and controlling the access to mastery ... impacts agency.

- ✦ What OM-related skillmaps live only in source experts ... as opposed to published documentation?
- ✦ Who controls access to the accumulated skillmaps [expertise] of OM?
- ✦ Which OM leaders, teachers, and pathfinders are encouraged to share their discoveries ... publicly and freely?

Controlling access to mastery is often used to create artificial (unnatural) shortages and chokepoints ... which are then leveraged – by a few – for a profit. That kind of system is often invested in maintaining an artificially constricted access to mastery.

Guidance for Somatic OMing & Mastery ...

Build [public] skills banks. Remove barriers to access and usability.

Make quality training, training standards, and training resources freely available.

Encourage public discussion – including publishing – of discoveries, standards, experiences, and problems.

Prioritize supporting and causing mastery at the level of community (CMLC) ... over causing mastery at the level of the individual. Focusing on the profiting of a few individuals over whole communities ... leads to information hoarding, artificially high prices[for access to mastery], shortages [of training and training resources], and systemic injustice.

* * *

Tribe & OM ::

What This Is ...

Tribe is the imagined, felt sense of belonging to one's communities.

How It Connects With Classic OM ...

OM is primarily a community-based practice. OMers thrive better in community and communication than they do in isolation, cut off from one another.

The old SensComm courses established an early set of community rituals for connection (a proto-8 Cups model) ... and nourishment / renewal. ("Everyone wants the same things ... to love and be loved, to see and be seen, to know one's purpose, and to feel connected....") These were intrinsic components of many Warehouse residents' OM practices. A key facet to many of the ritual communications ... was it was *equally* important to be able to see someone (for example) ... as it was to get one's own 'cup' of 'being seen' filled. Instead of the individualistic (and very western) value of ... "how do I get mine?" ... Classic OM teaches and supports a holistic / systemic approach: 1) "how do I get my cup [e.g., of 'approval'] filled? and 2) "how do I learn how to provide that service [i.e, that skillset] for others?" The community becomes richer ... and healthier ... when a *lot* of people are skilled in meeting core human needs.

A Guide to Somatic OMing

People often pursue sex ... as a substitute or placeholder for other [unfulfilled] needs ... including approval, connection, acknowledgement, basic touch, and [a sense of] belonging ... many of which require a community (other people) for fulfillment ... and most of which in modern western society have a dearth of socially approved rituals for fulfillment. OM begins a process of distinguishing, separating, and articulating (giving voice to) these "other" needs. Where mainstream culture is impoverished / parched ... OM culture can be hydrating / nourishing.

Guidance for Somatic OMing & the Tribe ...

You learn more and more quickly about OM and OMing ... in community (via either local or online communities).

Group OMing constitutes an advanced practice.

Group OMs have the *potential* to be a safer experience.

Communities can provide a wealth of unique perspectives to interpret new experiences ... and process them.

Rituals (shared social agreements) to meet a community's members' 8 Cups needs / desires can be created and shared. (The 8 Cups: approval, acknowledgement, connection, etc.)

The 8 Cups Metaphor for the Soma

The soma's natural landscape of desire can be represented by a metaphor called, 'the 8 Cups.'

Imagine that you have 8 cups ... Acknowledgement (to be seen), Expression (including play), Connection, Belonging, Intimacy (deep somatic rapport or resonance), Approval, Mastery (agency), and Pleasure (orgasm, in adults). The basic idea is each of these cups represents an instinctual, authentic, core, natural desire ... that will arise in every human ... and every child. Each person (beginning in childhood ... in age-appropriate ways) should be tasked with getting good at drinking from (receiving) and filling (providing) ... the contents ('strokes') from each 'cup.' So, for the Acknowledgement Cup ... some people may be 'stuck' ... because they either lack the ability to gracefully receive acknowledgement in public and let it in ... or they lack the ability to acknowledge others cleanly (aka, without deflection, undermining, or misdirection). As a member of the tribe, they are responsible for mastering both filling and drinking from that Cup. And it is in the tribe's best interest to ensure that members get 'unstuck' around *all* of the cups ... when one suffers, the whole tribe is unsettled / weakened.

(Someone who is weak around a given cup, say Acknowledgement, will often still work via the shadow (theirs and / or the tribe's) to get their 'fix' ... and that will lead to instances of 'placeholders' being used. That also leads to the whole ... "games within games" that dominate some social milieus ... as people strive to trick or manipulate others into fulfilling the particular need ... that they can't publicly 'own' – or get filled. In a word, they lack agency in the matter.)

Much of OM in the beginning is preoccupied with people ... beginning to detect, acknowledge, and tell the truth about *what* they desire ... instead of hiding everything (approval, acknowledgement, expression, basic touch, connection) under the generic label 'sex.'

The 8 Cups Model indicates a core set of social skills training that should be developed and made available to communities.

* * *

A Guide to Somatic OMing

Orgasm & OM ::

What This Is ...

In OM 'orgasm' is defined in a unique, nontraditional way. It works. Whereas orgasm is traditionally associated with the distinctly male act of climax / ejaculation ... in OM, orgasm is taken to be the whole of the wave ... that precedes, includes, and follows ... climax.

In the culture of OM, orgasm is energy ... and all [somatic] energy is seen as orgasmic. Alignment with, and openness to [a woman in] orgasm ... is the medium through which an OM practitioner reconnects to their body and restores a more natural dialogue with their intuitions, intuitive self, and their own deeper wisdom.

How It Connects With Classic OM ...

OM expands the definition of orgasm past the traditionally narrow focus on male climax.

OM offers a rich expanded somatic lexicon of distinctions within orgasm ... many of which are independently observable / verifiable during an OMer's practice.

The fundamental energy patterns and cycles of distinguished by OM's model of orgasm ... show up in other [nonsexual] areas of life. Many OM lessons transfer very nicely to 'normal' life.

Guidance for Somatic OMing & Orgasm ...

OM / orgasm is a gateway to numinous (energy-based) experiences.

A Guide to Somatic OMing

OM can be a gateway to a wealth of subtle and unique altered states / SAs (somatic addresses).

Learning to create, detect, and honor healthy social containers involving sex is a key skill and can foster integrity, good social habits, boundary management Best Practices, and a non-narcissistic self worthy of esteeming.

Pursuing / exploring orgasm via OM … can reveal many of the places you hide from yourself.

* * *

Numina & OM ::

What This Is ...

Numina is the sensed experience in the soma (body) of energy. It includes orgasm, but really is much broader than that ... encompassing other cross-cultural expressions like chi, prana, lifeforce, 'vibrancy,' and 'aliveness.'

How It Connects With Classic OM ...

OM is fundamentally an energy-based practice.

'Stroking the air above the clit' ... is one of the first introductions to OM as an energy-based practice.

Over time ... both strokee & stroker begin to develop their ability to detect energy (numina) ... and energy shifts, patterns, and cycles.

Learning how to 'read' one's own energy ... is key to self-alignment / integrity, full self-expression, being fully present, being centered, and powerful.

Guidance for Somatic OMing & Numina ...

OM is an energy-based practice.

Numina is a fancy word for energy. All orgasm is energy ... but not all energy is orgasm. The word numina is used to distinguish between the average person's understanding of 'energy' in human dynamics ... and OMers' use – and intricate awareness – of energy patterns. Basically, you can't talk to kids (and some adults) about orgasm ... but you can talk to them about numina (energy) patterns. It turns out that many of the energy patterns in OM have similar patterns ... in non-sexual contexts.

A Guide to Somatic OMing

"Follow the silver thread." In working with energy patterns and cycles, changes are often signaled by very subtle shifts in energy … detectable by the soma. Experienced OMers will often describe "following where energy wants to flow." That 'following' has also been described … as "following a silver [gossamer-like] thread …." Much of the personal attention and awareness development that occurs naturally over time in an OM practice … is a huge asset in detecting and following shifts in energy and energy patterns.

Numina can be partially understood … as an indicator of the energy of "feeling alive" (or 'numinosity').

Develop your connection to – and rapport with – your soma … and your ability to read energy and 'stroke' others – and yourself – energetically.

✳ ✳ ✳

Identity & OM ::

What This Is ...

Personal Identity is a dynamic, imagined construct originating in Mythos (stories) and represented ('embodied') in the Soma.

How It Connects With Classic OM ...

How one connects – or fails to connect – with orgasm ... plays a big role in one's self-identity

OM breaks old limiting models (stereotypes) about identity and what is possible. It can create over time ... an experience of personal identity as malleable and even fluid ... instead of fixed and rigid.

OMing re-introduces the concept of the soma (body) ... as an integral element ... in shaping one's personal identity. Instead of being discarded and scorned as irrelevant or merely an encumbrance ... the body / soma becomes the seed of a fascinating and endlessly rich trove of experiences, sensations, truths, and somatic addresses.

Identity is partially created ... out of a collection of stories ... about how *other people* can be. As we our partners open and flourish, it shifts our sense of what may be available ... for us. OM disrupts our old stories ... our old possibilities ... our old [somatic] destinations.

Guidance for Somatic OMing & Identity ...

We are not our public – or private – avatar [persona-mask].

Identity is by nature, fluid. Our modern culture [often] forces us to calcify ... our narratives about 'who *we* are.'

A Guide to Somatic OMing

Creating new mythos with new destinations and pathways ... together with adding new areas of mastery ... is an efficient way to rapidly shift / change / expand personal identity.

Each of the other 'domains' discussed above in this work also directly impact personal identity. All are potential gateways for change / expansion / self-improvement / creating something new.

* * *

A Guide to Somatic OMing

Planet & OM ::

What This Is ...

Planet is the baseline matrix defining and constraining [most] lifeforms.

How It Connects With Classic OM ...

By deepening our connection to soma – both ours and others' – OM restores our connection to the planet, the 'local domain' within which our biology arose and evolved. Our somas are – literally – integrated and interwoven with the biosphere of our planet.

Being in our soma – and in tune with our soma – can lead to more ethical and holistic choices and perspectives.

Guidance for Somatic OMing & Planet ...

Connect with others.

Build ethical somatic communities.

Create and make easily accessible ... skills banks with OM and essential social and communications skillmaps.

Tell the truth.

Support and CMLC (Cause Mastery at the Level of Community). Don't restrict or hoard expertise ... or restrict access to expertise: training, certification (public validation / verification), analysis, troubleshooting, and testing.

Support the restoration and recovery of the agency and expression of others – especially classically underserved demographic groups.

A Guide to Somatic OMing

Return to – and honor – the soma. If a proposed pathway / option overrides, damages, or weakens the soma ... it's not a solution. It's a fix ... and a costly one.

Design – and choose to play – clean [social] games ... that support the soma.

Humans have chaotic, contradictory, relatively primitive mythologies. Mythologies that frequently are at odds with supporting and nourishing their somas. Learn to build connections and relationships with other somas ... and mythologies that explain how to do that.

All somas are one soma ... whether human or critter ... we all start with some matrix of sensation and awareness. The personal details may be interesting ... but the commonalities are *breathtaking.*

All life specific to this planet ... is indelibly imprinted by *this* planet ... its gravity, magnetosphere, its solar and lunar cycles, its [bio]chemistry, its peculiar 'Goldilocks Zone.'

One planet ... one life ... one soma.

Connect.

* * *

:: WHAT'S NEXT ::

:: OM is a Political Act ::

"A woman has the right to have her clitoris stroked by a trained, willing partner of her choosing … and then get up, and go about her day … with no strings attached, owing nothing."

OMing can restore trust, rebuild rapport, and help recover and restore agency. All of these things are true.

And … OM is a political act.

OM is an act of rebellion against the patriarchy.

… it is a 'f*ck you' to everyone who advocates women should be seen and not heard, compliant, polite, eye candy, 'not too pushy / too vocal / too _____.'

Nicole Daedone may have created OM, OneTaste may have pushed OM out into the world with marketing and gimmicks, … but OM belongs to us … to the community. It's up to us to lead now.

* * *

A Guide to Somatic OMing

:: PATHS TO OMING ::

If you want to learn how to OM, here are some pathways (mileage may vary) …

- read the book, "Slow Sex," and dive in with a willing partner;
- read the book, "The 4-Hour Body," and dive in with a willing partner;
- learn from a willing – and patient – current *experienced* practitioner;
- take private lessons from a trained OM Coach;
- take a class in How to OM;
- be 'informally' coached by an experienced OMer;
- take Skype lessons from a trained OM Coach or experienced OMer;
- check out videos on OM and OMing on YouTube.

Other OM Options / Paths / Resources* ::

If you are interested in other OM-related resources, paths, and training, here are some worth looking into …

- "Slow Sex," by Nicole Daedone
- "The 4-Hour Body," by Tim Ferriss
- AASECT.org (lists accredited sex educators, coaches, & therapists)
- OneTaste OM Courses & OM Coaching
- The OMGYES! App
- Morehouse Courses (DOing was a precursor to OM)
- Welcomed Consensus Courses & Videos / DVDs
- YouTube Channels : ND + OT
- *alternative books …*
  - "Extended Massive Orgasm," by Steve Bodansky

A Guide to Somatic OMing

- "Women's Anatomy of Arousal," by Sheri Winston
- "Vagina," by Naomi Wolf
- "Pussy," by Regena Thomashauer
- "Finite & Infinite Games," and James Carse
- "The 5 Languages of Love," by Gary Chapman
- "Healing Sex," by Staci Haines
- "The Ethical Slut," by Janet W. Hardy and Dossie Easton
- "Ask: Building Consent Culture," by Kitty Stryker / Carol Queen
- "The Teacher's Shadow," by Alutha Jamancar
- "Light on Water," by Iona Eubanks
- "The Truth About Sex," by Gloria Brame
- "The Little Book of Energy Medicine," by Donna Eden
- "Stretching," by Bob Anderson
- "Female Ejaculation and the G Spot," by Deborah Sundahl
- "Mama Gena's School of Womanly Arts," by Regena Thomashauer
- "The Yoni Coloring Book," by H.L. Brooks
- "The Clitoral Truth," by Rebecca Chalker
- "Becoming Cliterate: Why Orgasm Equality Matters…," by Laurie Mintz
- "On Becoming an Alchemist," by Catherine MacCoun
- "A General Theory of Love," by Thomas Lewis
- "Language of Emotions," by Karla McLaren
- "Sensation: The New Science of Physical Intelligence," by Thalma Lobel
- "Social: Why Our Brains Are Wired to Connect," by Matthew D. Lieberman

- "Weaponized Lies: How to Think Critically in the Post-Truth Era," by Daniel J. Levitin
- "A Field Guide to Lies: Critical Thinking in the Information Age," by Daniel J. Levitin
- "Healing Trauma: Restoring the Wisdom of the Body," by Peter A. Levine
- "Sexual Healing: Transforming the Sacred Wound," by Peter A. Levine
- "Consciousness and the Social Brain," by Michael S.A. Graziano
- "Originals: How Non-Conformists Move the World," by Adam Grant
- "The Power of the Crone: Myths and Stories of the Wise Woman Archetype," by Clarissa Pinkola Estes
- "The Power of Myth," by Joseph Campbell
- "How Emotions Are Made: The Secret Life of the Brain," by Lisa Feldman Barrett
- "Cultures and Organizations: Software of the Mind," by Geert Hofstede
- "Exploring Culture: Exercises, Stories and Synthetic Cultures," by Gert Jan Hofstede
- "Tribes: We Need You to Lead Us," by Seth Godin
- "The E-Myth Revisited," by Michael Gerber
- "Sexual Outlaw, Erotic Mystic: The Essential Ida Craddock," by Vere Chappell
- "The Artist's Way," by Julia Cameron
- "The Body Has a Mind of Its Own," by Kate Reading
- "What Do Women Want?" by Daniel Bergner
- "The Art of Community: Building the New Age of Participation," by Jono Bacon

A Guide to Somatic OMing

- "Closer: Notes from the Orgasmic Frontier of Female Sexuality," by Sarah Barmak
- "Reality is Broken," by Jane McGonigal

Contact OneTaste and ask about current OM trainings, classes, or coaches that they can recommend.

(*Be warned the quality and integrity of OM training varies significantly currently. Caveat emptor.)

* * *

:: AFTERWORD ::

All advice is based on a description of the world, a model of the world, a mythology. Sometimes that description is personal and idiosyncratic, other times it arises from a shared, tribal description.

This work arises in part from the discoveries, adventures, and research others have shared with me – in particular, women ... and in part from my own unique journey. And it includes a new description of the world ... a new mythos ... that I have tinkering with for decades now.

As always when encountering a novel description of the world (and/or receiving advice) ... be curious, be skeptical, and, where appropriate, be playful. Bring your own experience, your own wisdom, your own intuitions ... and yes, your own legends, to your inquiry.

"Find a way. Find a balance. Discover who you are."

And when you are ready ... share your tales and adventures and learnings with the community.

* * *

A Guide to Somatic OMing

APPENDICES

:: A Clitoris Manifesto ::

01) "Stroke that Clit."

A woman has the right to have her clitoris stroked by a trained, willing partner of her choosing … and then get up, and go about her day … with no strings attached, owing nothing."

02) "Say It With Me: Vagina. Vagina. Vagina."

She has the unrestricted right to call her genitals (or any other part of her body) – in public – whatever she wants to: pussy, vagina, cunt, yoni.

03) #PussyArt

She has the [exclusive] right to take photos, make recordings, or create art … based on any and all parts of her body. She has the sole right to present (or license) those images as art, or personal expression, or as part of a declaration of political support or affinity.

04) "Who Has the Womb, Makes the Rules."

She has the right to full, unhindered access to birth control and healthcare.

05) "The Matriarchy Starts Here."

If she gives birth or chooses to become the guardian of a child, she has the right to full access to childcare and wellbeing services for her children and her chosen family.

06) "See Number 5."

She has the right to equal or greater payment for any services she performs, vis-a-vis, any other gender.

07) "Access to Mastery Impacts Agency."

She has the right to full and unencumbered access to skills banks containing the essential expertise (skillmaps / training) for a fully realized adult citizen: citizenry, financial, well-being, social networking, sexual agency, business ... among others.

08) "My Body, My Rules."

She has the exclusive right to offer any physical intimacy services / contact that use her body, attention, and expertise ... for money or for free. She has the right to offer (or market) those services, unencumbered, to any adult.

09) "Agency in Partnership."

She has the right to enter into an informal or formal partnership – including marriage – with an adult of any gender. And to leave that partnership – temporarily or permanently – at a time of her choosing. She has the right to extended – informal or formal – partnerships with more than one adult at a time.

* * *

"When women speak truly, they speak subversively."
— Ursula K. Le Guin

* * *

:: The Best OM Training Going Forward ::

Based on my experience and the reports I have received over the last decade, here are my recommendations for OM Training Best Practices.

1) Live OM Training

While prerequisites to learning how to OM may occur in a variety of formats, live OM coaching continues to be essential for many new OMers getting off to a good start in their OM practice.

Live OM coaching can occur in OM labs (after 'How to OM' classes), OM circles, or in private OM coaching sessions. It can be done by more seasoned OMers acting as *volunteer* guides or more formally trained professional OM coaches. Generally, guides or coaches who are seasoned women OMers are preferable.

2) The Establishment and Use of Phased OM Prerequisites

OM culture is rich and can be intense. Different training paths should be created to address differing knowledge gaps and / or values gaps in the prospective students … before they ever enter a 'How to OM' class.

Dumping people directly into a 'How to OM class is … unwise. Most people will have a range of questions and concerns that will need to be properly addressed *before* they enter the 'How to OM' class itself. Personal agency needs to better supported and honored. Under no circumstances should prospective students be 'coaxed' or pushed into taking the next class / prerequisite.

Screening, evaluation (both self-evaluation and evaluation by the training cadre caliber), and vetting (of both students and trainers / coaches) are all essential steps in the new era of OM.

A rich, "all-the-bells-and-whistles" OM training path should identified, tested, and refined, with care being taken to identify *all* of the areas that people have needed training and support in so far: communication fundamentals, ethics, personal agency, gendering, body mechanics, logistics, support for specific disabilities, etc. New students should be evaluated in the areas established to figure out what prerequisites they require – or are requesting – before taking *actual* OM courses. Actual OM trainings should occur by explicit mutual consent ... of the student *and* the trainer(s) – and at the initiative of the student only. Also ... under no circumstance should a trainer be pressured into accepting a student that is: outside the trainer's right range, underprepared, emotionally or ethically fragile, physically or mentally unwell, or just feels 'off' to them. (The practice is already edgy enough.)

Many of the identified prerequisites to OM can be met with online training videos / lectures, with careful followup around the main teaching points of each course. Some people will prefer – or need – live Q&A settings. And people should be encouraged to take courses as many times as they see fit. (Online versions should always be free, with no paywalls or email signups required.) Most of the content ... even of the prerequisites themselves ... will be edgy and emotionally charged for most people.

In the end, there should be a buffet of electives freely available to prep most prospective students to be able to answer the question ... "do I want to learn how to OM [with these people]?" ... from an informed position.

3) The Cultivation of Online Video Training & VR

OM communities, OM community coops, and OM coaches / trainers should take better advantage of online video platforms like YouTube and Vimeo.

A lot of the preparation for learning to OM can be handled in *OM-free* online courses ... for example, distinguishing desires & requests, sharing frames, ethics in gender-based communications, making clean requests ... can *all* be taught well in short, concise, well-planned videos ... *that do not once mention OM.* This is important because: 1) politics are getting messy and less exposure is sometimes prudent; 2) non-OMers can benefit from much of "pre-OM" training (aka, prerequisites); 3) you can easily create a customized list of YouTube links for specific people ... and have them watch them and come back to you with any questions.

Lastly, VR (virtual reality) tech promises to be a much less risky way for 'sensitive' explicit OM training ... to be communicated ... without actually "filming" anyone's pussy. It won't replace live OM coaching, but with a rich enough VR OM library ... it has the promise to eventually greatly reduce the need for live OM coaching. Eventually.

4) A Return to Women-Led Course Design

OM course design should almost always be led by women. A drive for a 'fifty-fifty' split (between women and men) is an attempt to powershare in an area where women's interests are paramount. It implies a weakness and neediness about men. Choose male allies who are confident enough to play a supporting role ... in an area where women's voices are quite naturally and rightly prominent – women's orgasm.

Additionally, in most arenas where there is a fifty-fifty split between women and men in leadership ... as a result of cultural conditioning (of all sexes) ... the men end up with a dominant share of bandwidth, airtime, and attention. This was painfully illustrated in the recent OT co-presidency: a man and a woman were co-Presidents of OT for a spell. During that time, the man made most of the 'public' announcements. He became the de facto public face for the organization. The woman took essentially second position. Both people should have known better. Men who insist on a 50-50 power split ... misunderstand –

A Guide to Somatic OMing

and overinflate – their position (and importance) in a shifting world of gender fluidity. Straight men were never at a 50% share in a world that is truly LBGQT-aware. Don't encourage bad habits.

Women: lead. OM is your house.

5) Focus on Developing & Supporting Volunteer-Based OM Training

Volunteer-based OM training should be supported by almost all OM communities. Commercial OM training has too often sold out ethics and morals for profit – or for just a desperate attempt to stay afloat. People should never be considered 'marks' – that goes even more so for people wanting to explore OM and connection.

The 'wealth' of OM communities may be best measured in how much expertise they possess … and how much they have unrestricted access to. Crush the marketing gimmick of 'fear-of-missing-out' (FOMO). It denigrates people and weakens and hijacks personal agency. Businesses which depend on it to make payroll should be shuttered.

Communities can support volunteer-based OM training by … sharing community expertise and learnings freely (while ensuring privacy and anonymity) … by holding community OM Days, discussing issues that arise in community, producing PG-rated OM-related (but OM-free) trainings online (via YouTube), and generally, helping OMers tell their stories – light and dark.

6) Course Design Transparency & Standardization

Avoiding publicizing the design, structure, and content of your OM courses is way to avoid accountability and responsibility. Not knowing what exactly is being offered in a proposed course undermines the prospective student's ability to make a choice in their best interest. It undermines and dilutes their personal agency.

OM trainers, teachers, and coaches should move to a public OM model – and publish a code of conduct / ethics – that they can be held accountable for.

For too many years, OM course design was randomly and haphazardly generated – all under the safety net of being "experimental." OM is 14 years old this year. It's past time for its leaders and teachers to grow up.

If [new] OM courses are going to be offered, actually 'design' them – and then publish your design, for other OM practitioners to discuss and critique. And improve on. It's a meditation practice. It is not quantum computing chip design. No one is ever going to make a ton of money teaching a meditation practice. Start working in community … instead of desperately barricading you and your one 'special' idea … from the community.

7) Shift Course Design & Endorsement from Corporate to Community-Led Coops

Until now, most OM training and OM course design has been produced as commercial products by a handful of corporations and businesses. Over time, that needs to shift to community-led and community-run cooperatives (coops).

These coops need to start initiating OM course designs – not for profit, but sourced by coop-trained volunteers.

It is also time to look at the process of endorsing and sanctioning OM Model changes and variations. OT 'certified' a *lot* of OM coaches over the years … but each new coaching program varied – sometimes widely – in what they were 'taught' and were certified in. Even today, there are no clear lists as to what each 'class' of coaches was actually taught – and how much of what they were taught has been discarded … and is no longer 'sanctioned.' Again … the personal agency of students seeking specific coaching is undercut … if their coach can't actually establish *what* they were trained in.

A Guide to Somatic OMing

Over time, for OM to truly thrive ... communities – probably through coops – will need to take on endorsing / sanctioning OM course designs.

* * *

:: About the Author ::

My name is Alutha Zatoichi Jamancar.

My OMing experience began in April 2006. I was a full-time Warehouse resident from July 2006 til July 2008. The Warehouse was a women-led community of 40+ OMers collectively researching women's orgasm. I completed or assisted in more then a dozen OM-related courses over those 2 years. I was the first person not in the original leadership core to be asked to be BOH (back-of-the-house). I completed over 2000 OMs in those 2 years. I also had more than 6 research partners in that time.

I was a member of the semi-public online OMing community called the Chatboard from 2006 til its closure. I have been a member of 3 versions of the OM Hub (another online community of OMers), as well as several other prominent independent online OM communities. I have posted extensively over the years on OM and OMing, and have been coached – both live and online – by Nicole Daedone, her core staff, and my research partners. I was also one of the only Warehouse residents to publicly call out Nicole when I thought she was 'off.' I produced two of the three Warehouse Era podcasts distributed by PLM.

I am known in the OM community as an advocate and a fan of OM.

I have been advocating for ethical training business standards & reforms for OM-related businesses for over a decade.

I created and contributed over 90% of the posts to the OM Report Facebook Page, one of the first independent OM platforms.

I created a (free) online OM Lexicon and populated it with over 200 entries.

I am also a man and I am writing about OM ... a woman-centric practice. So my direct experience of OM is as a stroker. Any information about the strokee's

A Guide to Somatic OMing

experience that I gathered over the years ... was provided – generously – by women OMers.

What I have learned about OM is a direct result of women patiently teaching me, starting with the creation and sharing of the OM Model by Nicole Daedone. Women – a lot of women – have shaped and molded my OM practice. In group OMs, women I've never met before made me a little bit wiser ... through the direct (and indirect) transmission of their OM practice. Even the men who shared information and discoveries ... did so because they OMed with – and learned from – women. As a result, I have a ton of info on OMing I have accumulated over the years. Some information is about Classic OM and some is about deeper patterns and resonances within OM that I noticed over time.

I consider OM to be the purview of women.

In the years since the first book on OM, "Slow Sex" by Nicole Daedone, was released, I had hoped that a woman writer-leader would step up and write in more detail – and in book form – on the practice of OM, but between the founder of OM (Nicole Daedone) selling OneTaste a few years ago and retiring from teaching ... and the absence – and very understandable reticence, given the current political climate – of anyone arising to a public leadership position in the next wave of OM teachers and trainers ... I have decided now is the time to get some version of what I have accumulated out into the world.

So ... from women ... to me ... to you.

As a result, you will find some info on Classic OM in this work. And some info about what I am calling Somatic OMing – which draws on my own lessons and models on OMing. Neither body of knowledge is complete. But people should have access to the lessons I and others have accrued ... in order to discuss, and try out ... in their own OM practice.

OM is fundamentally a community-based practice.

A Guide to Somatic OMing

This is what I have to contribute to the global OM community ... today.

* * *

:: The Design of This Book ::

Manuscript Pipeline ::

This book was first crafted online, through a series of posts, notes, and blog entries … primarily on Facebook. This ensures that my work has the widest possible public (and free) access.

The resulting draft was first reformatted for release as an ebook in the Amazon Kindle format. (See KDP.com for more info.)

Next, the draft will be reformatted again for release in paperback format. (See KDP.com for info on self-publishing options.)

Releasing my online book in ebook and paperback formats allows me to monetize my work … while keeping the content freely accessible in online notes (which are hard to read in long doses, but serviceable).

Offline, I primarily used Apple Notes and TextEdit to prep my initial posts, and Apple Pages to generate the print-ready PDF for the paperback edition.

Art Design ::

Colors ...

The cover has 4 basic colors: orange, a reddish-brown, white, and bright red. I use this color scheme for other OM-related works.

The orange represents a (non-caucasian / nonwhite) skin color.

The reddish-brown represents the darker pigments of a woman's labia.

The white is used for high contrast.

The bright red color represents the engorgement of the clitoris and pussy lips.

Glyphs ...

I use two basic glyphs: a box with a circle and 3 dashes, and a circle containing a human-like figure.

I chose the box glyph to represent an OM. The rectangle represents the OM container, the 3 dashes ... strokes in an OM, and the 'O' represents the woman's orgasm.

I chose the circle glyph to represent a woman's body ... her soma. The tiny triangle at the center represents her clit.

In the front cover design, one of the rectangles is bright red. This is done to represent the deeper practice of Somatic OMing.

Cover Layout ...

I used OmniGraffle 6.6 to create the cover art for the Kindle ebook edition and the paperback edition.

* * *

:: The Desire & Request Distinction ::

Desire and Request: Expanding Choice and Consciousness in Relationship

****

Most people in romantic or sensuous relationships in this country [the U.S.] have the distinction (or difference) between 'speaking a desire of theirs' and 'making a request to fulfill that desire' collapsed.

****

What I discovered in my research one year with my lover was that when she had a desire in her body *and* spoke that desire congruent with what was in her body (no weakening, soft-pedaling, or cloudy speech), the alignment caused a pleasurable release in my body and in hers. And this, without actually acting on the desire!

A key piece was separating out … that she had a desire and was communicating what that desire was … from her actually making a request to fulfill that desire.

Without that separation, quite of bit of juggling goes on in her head as she frantically evaluates whether I am going to 'spontaneously' act on her spoken desire … and whether she approves of that or not … *and* whether she approves of approving of that or not!

So I created that speaking the desire is not a request. This proved enormously beneficial to both of us. She could concentrate on simply telling her truth … speaking her desire congruent to what she felt in her body … with no obligation / expectation by either of us to act on it. And I no longer had to:

- figure out what her desire was;
- figure out whether she was telling me the truth or not;
- figure out whether she was lying to herself about her desire;

- figure out whether I wanted to fulfill her desire in that instant;
- figure out whether she expected me to fulfill her desire in that instant;
- figure out whether – if I fulfilled her desire – she would punish me or approve of me.

A big part of the reason that many women do not speak their desires is this cloud of calculations needs to be navigated, and it can be *very* intimidating. So instead they want a partner who will simply intuitively *know* what they want without the women speaking it.

Distinguishing this created a huge opening for connection with my lover. My job became very simple:
Notice what my body felt before she stated her desire and after.

Read whether or not she had spoken her desire powerfully, fully, and truthfully. Support her in bringing her truth (true desire) forth.

That meant no poaching on the spoken desire, by *sweetly* and wordlessly beginning to fulfill it. And finding a way to approve of her desire without giving up my ability later to choose 'yes' or 'no' to a request (from her) to fulfill that desire.

Once that is done, I have heard her desires. I know that they are hers. I am clear on what they are. And if she makes an explicit request of me to fulfill a desire later, she is taking responsibility for her turn-on, she is in her power. I have an access to fulfilling her desire and receiving her approval. And that means she doesn't need to hide herself or her turn-on, and I can be fearless with her.

Speaking a desire is not the same as making a request. Collapsing these two is the source of a kind of mashing practiced by both sexes.

* * *

A Guide to Somatic OMing

:: OM Lexicon ::

I have created an online OM Lexicon with ever 200+ entries, which can be found at https://tinyurl.com/y7okmhf2 or https://www.facebook.com/notes/little-book-of-om/om-lexicon-page-2-of-3-v-4/1042092605941016/.

* * *

Made in the USA
Las Vegas, NV
07 August 2021